Hypoxia: Mechanisms and Effects

Hypoxia: Mechanisms and Effects

Edited by Ronin Wahlberg

hayle
medical

New York

Hayle Medical,
750 Third Avenue, 9th Floor,
New York, NY 10017, USA

Visit us on the World Wide Web at:
www.haylemedical.com

ISBN: 978-1-63241-882-1

Cataloging-in-Publication Data

Hypoxia : mechanisms and effects / edited by Ronin Wahlberg.
    p. cm.
Includes bibliographical references and index.
ISBN 978-1-63241-882-1
1. Anoxemia. 2. Oxygen in the body. 3. Oxygen--Physiological effect. I. Wahlberg, Ronin.
RC103.A4 H96 2020
616.2--dc23

Table of Contents

Preface..VII

Chapter 1   **Interplay between Hypoxia, Inflammation and Adipocyte Remodeling in
the Metabolic Syndrome**..1
Ana Marina Andrei, Anca Berbecaru-Iovan, Felix Rareş Ioan Din-Anghel,
Camelia Elena Stănciulescu, Sorin Berbecaru-Iovan, Ileana Monica Baniţă and
Cătălina Gabriela Pisoschi

Chapter 2   **Hypoxia-Induced Molecular and Cellular Changes in the Congenitally
Diseased Heart: Mechanisms and Strategies of Intervention** 27
Dominga Iacobazzi, Massimo Caputo and Mohamed T Ghorbel

Chapter 3   **Hypoxia and its Emerging Therapeutics in Neurodegenerative, Inflammatory and
Renal Diseases** 43
Deepak Bhatia, Mohammad Sanaei Ardekani, Qiwen Shi and Shahrzad Movafagh

Chapter 4   **Stage-Specific Effects of Hypoxia on Interstitial Lung Disease**....................84
Sandeep Artham and Payaningal R. Somanath

Chapter 5   **Adaptations to Chronic Hypoxia Combined with Erythropoietin Deficiency in
Cerebral and Cardiac Tissues**...104
Raja El Hasnaoui-Saadani

Chapter 6   **Epigenetic Programming of Cardiovascular Disease by Perinatal Hypoxia and
Fetal Growth Restriction**..121
Paola Casanello, Emilio A. Herrera and Bernardo J. Krause

Chapter 7   **Hypoxic Upregulation of ARNT (HIF-1β): A Cell-Specific Attribute with
Clinical Implications** 140
Markus Mandl and Reinhard Depping

Chapter 8   **Role of the Hypoxia-Inducible Factor in Periodontal Inflammation** 155
Xiao Xiao Wang, Yu Chen and Wai Keung Leung

Permissions

List of Contributors

Index

Preface

It is often said that books are a boon to mankind. They document every progress and pass on the knowledge from one generation to the other. They play a crucial role in our lives. Thus I was both excited and nervous while editing this book. I was pleased by the thought of being able to make a mark but I was also nervous to do it right because the future of students depends upon it. Hence, I took a few months to research further into the discipline, revise my knowledge and also explore some more aspects. Post this process, I begun with the editing of this book.

Hypoxia is the condition in which there is a deprivation in the supply of oxygen in the body or a region of the body. It occurs when there is a reduction in oxygen pressure below the normal range. However, it can be a part of the normal physiology, and may occur with strenuous physical exercise or during hypoventilation training. It may be generalized or local. Generalized hypoxia can be a high-altitude disease or one in which a mixture of gases with low oxygen content has been inhaled. Fatigue, nausea, numbness and cerebral anoxia are some common symptoms. Hypoxia can result in cyanosis when severe and tissues may become gangrenous. Such tissue hypoxia may be due to low cardiac output, low hemoglobin concentration and low hemoglobin saturation. This book provides comprehensive insights into the mechanisms and effects of hypoxia. It will also provide interesting topics for research, which interested readers can take up. With state-of-the-art inputs by acclaimed experts in pulmonology, this book targets students and professionals.

I thank my publisher with all my heart for considering me worthy of this unparalleled opportunity and for showing unwavering faith in my skills. I would also like to thank the editorial team who worked closely with me at every step and contributed immensely towards the successful completion of this book. Last but not the least, I wish to thank my friends and colleagues for their support.

Editor

Interplay between Hypoxia, Inflammation and Adipocyte Remodeling in the Metabolic Syndrome

Ana Marina Andrei, Anca Berbecaru-Iovan,

Felix Rareş Ioan Din-Anghel,

Camelia Elena Stănciulescu, Sorin Berbecaru-Iovan,

Ileana Monica Baniță and Cătălina Gabriela Pisoschi

Abstract

Obesity, a major social and health problem in many countries, is due to the accumulation of white adipose tissue in subcutaneous and visceral depots. The discovery of adipocytes capacity of synthesis of numerous adipocytokines and growth factors and the cross talk between adipocytes and cells of the adipose stromo-vascular fraction had highlighted the role of adipose tissue dysfunction in obesity. In visceral obesity the unbalanced synthesis of pro- and anti-inflammatory adipocytokines contributes to the development of the metabolic syndrome which cumulates the factors that increase the risk for ischemic heart disease and cerebral stroke. Adipose tissue accumulation is associated with a state of chronic inflammation, and local hypoxia is considered its underlying cause due to the hypertrophic or/and the hyperplasic growth of the fat pad. Adipose tissue hypoxia is one of the first pathophysiological changes and was placed as a missing link between obesity and low-grade inflammation present in the metabolic syndrome. Hypoxia is a major trigger for adipose tissue remodeling including adipocyte death, inflammation, tissue fibrosis, and angiogenesis. Recently, the role of hypoxia in brown adipose tissue dysfunction, a tissue presumed as the biologic counterbalance of the metabolic disturbances in human obesity, is discussed.

Keywords: adipose tissue, hypoxia, inflammation, metabolic syndrome, fibrosis, angiogenesis

1. Introduction

Until two decades ago, the adipose tissue has been considered one of the least dynamic structures of the mammalian organism involved exclusively in fat storage. Some key events have changed this mechanistic point of view, and now the whole fat of an organism is viewed as a complex organ composed of at least two main varieties of adipose tissues: the white adipose tissue (WAT) containing unilocular adipocytes and the brown adipose tissue (BAT) formed by multilocular adipocytes. Besides this different type of adipocytes, both tissues contain a non-adipocitary stromo-vascular fraction that includes undifferentiated cells, preadipocytes, fibroblasts, inflammatory cells, and various amounts of vessels and nerves. The adult adipose organ is divided into two types of depots: subcutaneous/peripheral and visceral/central constituted of lobules of unilocular adipocytes sustained by the stromo-vascular fraction well vascularized and innervated [1–5].

A significant development in the knowledge of adipose tissue is related to its function as an endocrine organ, both types of tissues being able to elaborate adipocytokines, humoral factors with various metabolic, vascular, pro-inflammatory, and anti-inflammatory roles [2, 4].

The accumulation of WAT in physiological depots leads to obesity characterized by an increase of the body mass index (BMI) over 30 kg/m^2 [6]. Obesity became a major social and health problem in many countries (between one quarter and one third of the population), a recent report of the World Health Organization (WHO) mentioning more than 1.9 billion of adult overweight subjects worldwide, more than 600 millions being obese [7]. From a pathogenically point of view, the quality and the distribution of adipose tissue seem to be more important in triggering the metabolic syndrome than the quantity of the fat per se. A direct relationship is accepted between abdominal/visceral fat accumulation—apple-shaped obesity—and the emergence and development of the metabolic syndrome or abdominal and pelvic cancers. Unbalanced synthesis of pro- and anti-inflammatory adipocytokines in visceral obesity contributes to the development of many features of the metabolic syndrome which cumulates the factors that increase the risk for ischemic heart disease and cerebral stroke: apple-shaped fat deposition, impaired glucose metabolism, dyslipidemia, and high blood pressure [8–10]. Pear-shaped obesity—i.e., subcutaneous fat accumulation—has a minimal risk for the development of such pathologies even at the same BMI greater than 30 kg/m^2 [11–13].

Hypoxia is one of the mechanisms responsible for the development of the metabolic changes and the pro-inflammatory milieu of white adipose tissue in obesity [3].

Tissue partial O$_2$ pressure (pO$_2$) reflects the balance between O$_2$ delivery and consumption, and continuous, chronic low O$_2$ tension occurs as a tissue inability to provide adequate compensatory vascular supply [3, 14, 15]. Obviously, adipose tissue hypoxia has a polymorphic feature since it depends on the adipose tissue blood flow regulation, different between the adipose phenotype WAT or BAT, the adipose fat pad localization, subcutaneous or visceral, and the delay of time between the onset of hypoxia and its quantification.

In healthy lean young adult, the pO$_2$ in adipose tissue is considered 55–60 mm Hg [14, 16] similar to the general tissue oxygenation [4], but important differences were reported in obese subjects. Oxygen supply was found markedly lower (44.7 mm Hg) in obese subjects in fasting and postprandial status than in lean subjects (55.4 mmHg) [14, 17], but Goossens et al. [18] found that in WAT of obese subjects the pO_2 was even higher (67.4 mmHg) than lean (46.8 mmHg). Of note, the pO_2 is not in a direct relation with the surface of the vascular network in the adipose pad. Capillary density for both subcutaneous and visceral depots is lower in obese human than in lean, but in lean subjects, the density is greater in visceral location [14, 19]. Even if BAT adipose tissue is more vascularized than WAT, it was indicated that obesity also causes BAT hypoxia, the same response being noted in multilocular adipocytes that became larger in obese animals [20]. Interestingly, BAT hypoxia seems to be temperature-dependent. Xue et al. proved that there is no hypoxia in mice housed at 30°C, but it appears in animals living at 4°C [21].

Adipose tissue is one of the most plastic organs in adults gifted with the ability of a continuous remodeling—extends or regresses depending on nutrient intake. The plasticity of any tissue is due to its capacity of extending vasculature which requires the cross talk between adipocytes and stromal and endothelial cells in the case of adipose tissue.

There are several arguments in favor of this "hypoxia concept." Normally, each adipocyte is surrounded by capillaries, and it is widely accepted that WAT is poorly oxygenated in obese individuals because adipocytes may be up to 200 μm, so larger than the normal diffusion distance of oxygen within tissues. As adipose tissue mass rapidly increases, clusters of unilocular adipocyte distance from the vessels and pockets of hypoxia are generated [22]. Another cause presumed for adipose tissue hypoxia is the loss of endothelial cells usually associated with the damage of parenchymal cells in other tissues. Recently, the interest in brown adipose tissue (BAT) increased, and studies have indicated that obesity determines also BAT hypoxia and the loss of its thermogenic capacity [20].

Chronic adipose tissue hypoxia has been suggested to be part of the pathogenesis of adipocyte dysfunction [14, 23, 24]. Local hypoxia triggers the generation of reactive oxygen species (ROS) and endoplasmic reticulum (ER) stress [25] and initiates the inflammatory response able to regulate the balance between angiogenic factors and inhibitors in order to stimulate angiogenesis and increase blood flow. The paucity of endothelial barrier is associated with the release of profibrogenic and pro-inflammatory cytokines and an augmented influx of inflammatory cells [26]. There is considerable evidence that obese adipose tissue is markedly infiltrated with macrophages which participate in the inflammatory pathways and are very important in adipose tissue remodeling, macrophage infiltration being signalized by lipid-overloaded adipocytes necrosis. Numerous reports emphasized that visceral adipose tissue in obese individuals is more fibrotic than that of lean subjects [27–29].

Normally, BAT and WAT produce various pro-angiogenic factors and cytokines able to induce remodeling of the vasculature, and as a response to hypoxia, an unbalanced production of these multiple bioactive pro-angiogenic and antiapoptotic growth factors synthesized by the adipose stromal cells may occur. Local hypoxia in obese is the underlying cause of an increase of macrophage cell number accompanied by the state of chronic inflammation and impaired adipokine secretion. Hypoxia promotes the delivery of many adipocytokines related to inflammation and tissue remodeling needed for angiogenesis to the ischemic tissue, such as macrophage migration inhibitory factor (MIF), granulocyte-macrophage colony-stimulating factor (GM-CSF), matrix metalloproteinases MMP-2 and MMP-9, transforming growth factor (TGF)-β, vascular endothelial growth factor (VEGF), interleukins (IL-1, IL-6, IL-10), tumor necrosis factor (TNF)-α, angiopoietin-like (Angptl)-4, and leptin [4, 15, 22, 30–32].

This chapter summarizes the potential links between hypoxia, inflammation, adipocyte hypertrophy, and macrophage infiltration of adipose tissue and the effects of inflammatory mediators on its remodeling.

2. Essentials of adipose organ structure and functions

The adult adipose organ is composed by two types of adipose depots divided into adipose lobules of (i) unilocular adipose tissue (WAT—white adipose tissue) composed of unilocular cells and (ii) brown adipose tissue (BAT), formed by multilocular adipocytes (**Figure 1a** and **b**).

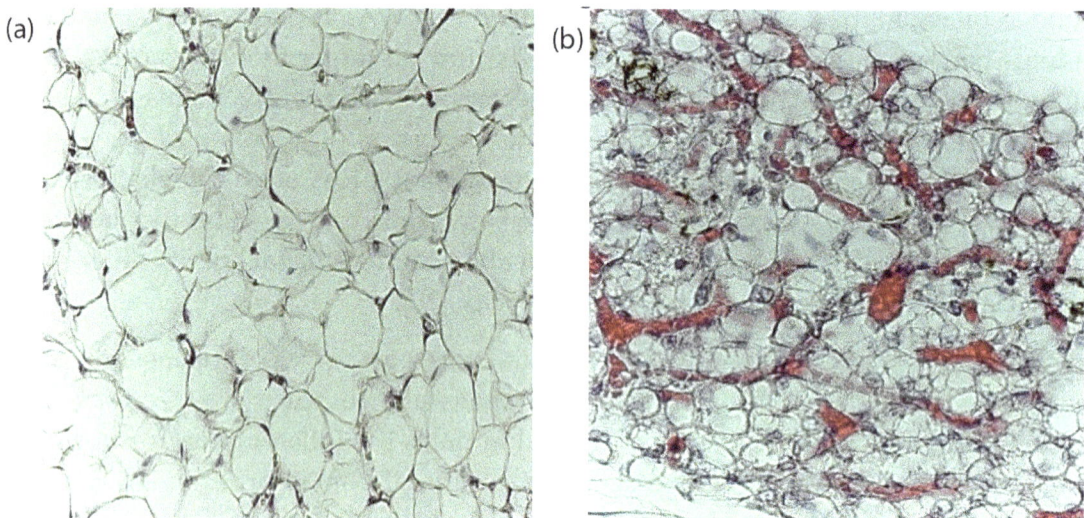

Figure 1. (a) Human adult subcutaneous WAT (hematoxylin and eosin staining, ob. ×40) and (b) human newborn visceral adipose depot with unilocular WAT and multilocular BAT adipocytes (hematoxylin and eosin staining, ob. ×20).

Both types of cells organized into adipose lobules are sustained by the stromo-vascular fraction well vascularized and innervated [11, 33]. Anatomically, WAT depots are located primarily in two major areas—subcutaneous/peripheral and visceral/central, which differ in the composition of the stromo-vascular fraction [34, 35]. Although at a first view the adipose tissue looks quite simple, a deeper molecular analysis revealed a high heterogeneity of cells. With respect to adipose cells, recent research identified both in rodent and men, the third type of adipocytes with common features of WAT and BAT adipocytes named "brite" or "beige" cells.

BAT, so named because of its yellow-brown color in vivo due to a very rich vascularization, is distinguishable morphologically from WAT by its cytoplasmic multiple droplets of stored triglycerides, while WAT contains a single large droplet. The multilocular cells are rich in mitochondria containing the uncoupling protein (UCP)1 which is uniquely present in BAT and therefore considered a marker for it (**Figure 2**).

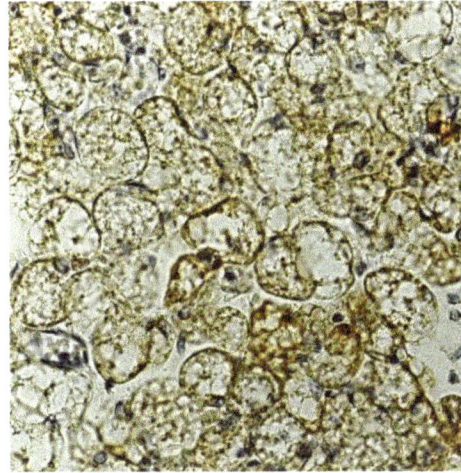

Figure 2. Newborn human brown adipocytes labeled with UCP1 (IHC, ob. ×40).

In humans, two types of BAT are present: (i) the classical (or constitutive BAT—cBAT) that is fully developed at birth and then reduced to remain in human adult only in a symmetrical cervical position and around the clavicles as very recently localized by PET/CT scanning, and the second type of brown adipocytes named "beige" or "brite" (brown in white), inducible or recruitable BAT (rBAT). This is composed of isolated brown multilocular cells resident between white cells mainly in subcutaneous depots [36, 37]. WAT is recognized as the site of fat storage, while BAT acts, as in rodents, as a heat-generating tissue through uncoupled oxidative phosphorylation which involves the action of UCP1 [38].

The functional complexity of adipose tissue is also due to the heterogeneity of cell phenotypes located in the non-adipocitary stromo-vascular fraction that includes undifferentiated or mesenchymal cells, preadipocytes, fibroblasts, and inflammatory cells (macrophages, lymphocytes, and mast cells). These cells are surrounded by a very complex network of vessels and nerves. The vascular network is more developed and branched in BAT than in WAT [39]. Normal metabolic functions and their imbalance involve a cross talk between adipocytes and the cells from the stromo-vascular fraction mediated by the components of adipose tissue extracellular matrix (ECM).

WAT secretoma. The discovery of leptin by Friedman in 1994 initiated the recognition of white adipocytes as major endocrine cells that secrete numerous bioactive molecules: lipids (such as free fatty acids mobilized in lipolysis, prostaglandins, and endocannabinoids) and proteins (termed "adipokines" or "adipocytokines" with metabolic and pro-/anti-inflammatory functions) [40]. Several adipocytokines are listed in **Table 1**. Impaired production of adipokines is associated with the pathogenesis of obesity-related disorders—type 2 diabetes mellitus, metabolic syndrome, cardiovascular diseases, and certain types of cancer [2, 41–44]. Generally, blood adipocytokine levels rise with the increase of fat mass except for adiponectin and omentin levels which are reported to be lower in obese and overweight subjects [31, 45, 46].

Adipocytokine	Function
Leptin	Feeding behavior, fat mass, pro-angiogenic
Adiponectin	Insulin sensitivity, anti-inflammatory, pro-angiogenic
Resistin	Insulin resistance, pro-inflammatory, antiangiogenic
Visfatin (pre-B-cell colony-enhancing factor, PBEF)	Insulin resistance, pro-inflammatory
Vaspin (visceral adipose tissue-derived serpin)	Insulin resistance
Omentin	Insulin resistance
Retinol-binding protein (RBP)-4	Insulin resistance
Serum amyloid A	Insulin resistance, pro-inflammatory
Cholesteryl ester transfer protein (CETP)	Lipid metabolism
Lipoprotein lipase (LPL)	Lipid metabolism
Adipocyte fatty acid-binding protein (A-FABP)-4	Lipid metabolism
Perilipin	Lipid metabolism
Apelin	Vasodilatation, pro-angiogenic
Angiotensinogen	Regulation of blood pressure
Angiotensin II	Regulation of blood pressure
Adipsin (adipocyte trypsin/complement factor D)	Lipid and glucose metabolism, inflammation
Tumor necrosis factor (TNF)-α	Pro-inflammatory
Interleukin 6 (IL-6)	Pro-inflammatory
C-reactive protein (CRP)	Pro-inflammatory
Plasminogen activator inhibitor (PAI)-1	Fibrinolysis, pro-angiogenic
Monocyte chemoattractant protein (MCP)-1	Macrophage activation
Intercellular adhesion molecule (ICAM)-1	Macrophage activation
Fibroblast growth factor (FGF)-2	Pro-angiogenic
Hepatocyte growth factor (HGF)	Pro-angiogenic
Platelet-derived growth factor (PDGF)	Pro-angiogenic
Vascular endothelial growth factor (VEGF)	Pro-angiogenic
Transforming growth factor (TGF)-β	Inflammation, fibrosis
Matrix metalloproteinases (MMPs)	Pro- and antiangiogenic, ECM remodeling
Tissue inhibitor of metalloproteinases (TIMPs)	Antiangiogenic, ECM remosdeling

Table 1. Adipocytokines and their main biological effects (adapted with permission from [31]).

Leptin and adiponectin are the most important hormones secreted by white adipocytes with multiple metabolic roles (regulating appetite and energy balance, insulin sensitivity) but also encompass angiogenic and anti-inflammatory actions [2, 4]. Leptin increases the vascular permeability in adipose tissue and influences microvessels density [47].

Adiponectin is regarded as a link between obesity and related metabolic disorders because it improves glucose and lipid metabolism and prevents inflammation [15]. There are many other members of the "adipokinome" involved in the inflammatory response: tumor necrosis factor (TNF)-α, interleukins (IL-6, IL-8, IL-10), monocyte chemoattractant protein (MCP)-1, and macrophage migration inhibitory factor (MIF) [4, 15, 22]. Besides the adipocytes, many other cells from the stromo-vascular fraction secrete inflammatory cytokines and chemokines in response to adipocyte hypertrophy or hypoxic conditions. Other adipokines related to inflammation include several crucial angiogenic factors, such as vascular endothelial growth factor (VEGF), hepatocyte growth factor (HGF)-1, angiopoetin-2, nerve growth factor (NGF), plasminogen activator inhibitor (PAI)-1, apelin, and adipsin [4, 30–32]. The release of numerous inflammatory adipocytokines is markedly increased in obesity-related diseases. Subcutaneous and visceral adipose tissue display differences in their adipokinome. Even if the results of in vitro and in vivo studies are controversial, it can be assumed, for example, that leptin and adiponectin are mainly produced in vivo by the subcutaneous adipocytes, while others (angiotensinogen, A-fatty acid-binding protein (FABP)-4, IL-6) are secreted at higher levels in visceral adipose tissue [48–51].

3. Adipose tissue dysfunction and hypoxia

Adipocyte capacity of synthesis corroborated with the clinical observation that a proportion of obese individuals seem to be protected against metabolic syndrome [52] had highlighted the role of adipose tissue dysfunction in obesity. Obesity is so long considered a genetic predisposition that promotes the excess of energy intake or the scarce energy expenditure.

In humans, the adipose tissue from the two main locations (subcutaneous and visceral) shows anatomical and functional differences (in contrast to subcutaneous adipose tissue, abdominal depots drain directly onto the portal circulation [31]) and different gene expressions.

Oxygen is a main nutritional factor without which oxidation of nutrients in aerobic tissues cannot take place. The decrease of oxygen level in various tissues can occur even if the total amount provided to the organism is not reduced [20]. Evinced hypoxia that follows low oxygen tension has numerous implications for cellular metabolism and transcriptional program [27]. Recent research suggests that adipose tissue hypoxia occurs in obese mice and even in human subjects. In obese rodents the existence of hypoxia was demonstrated by qualitative reaction (using hypoxic cell markers, such as pimonidazole—PIMO) or quantitative technique using needle-type oxygen sensors [3, 15, 22, 23]. In human obese subjects, the results are more controversial since normoxia and even hyperoxia have been reported in various experiments [18, 20, 53].

Chronic hypoxia has been suggested to be part of the pathogenic pathways leading to adipose tissue dysfunction [14, 23, 24].

Local hypoxia triggers the main alterations defining the adipose tissue dysfunction: generation of ROS and oxidative stress [54], ER stress [25], adipocyte death [55], inhibition of adiponectin expression [55, 56], and leptin hyperproduction [57] and initiates the inflammatory response able to regulate the balance between angiogenic and inhibitor factors in order to stimulate angiogenesis and increase blood flow.

More causes of adipose tissue hypoxia are discussed, this concept being related to the histological changes of the adipose obese tissue—hyperplasia and adipocyte hypertrophy. Reduction of blood supply in adipose pads is a common mechanism of tissue hypoxia. Reduced adipose tissue blood flow in obese rats and humans was reported many years ago (Larsen et al, 1966, West et al., 1987 cited by [26]), being associated with insulin resistance in obese individuals [17, 18]. Adipose tissue angiogenesis is insufficient to maintain normoxia in the growing number of fat-storing cells in adipose depots as they are in obesity. Histological analysis has demonstrated a scarce capillary network in abdominal subcutaneous depots in obese subjects compared to the leans [14, 18].

A second cause is related to the increased size of adipocytes—hypertrophy—reaching in obese subjects a diameter larger than 150–200 μm [45]. This exceeds the normal capacity of oxygen diffusion through the tissue (100–200 μm), and oxygenation of adipose tissue will be compromised [58].

Hypoxia-inducible factor (HIF)-1 is the key transcriptional factor involved in response to hypoxia, which moves into the nucleus and binds to hypoxia-response elements from a myriad of target genes to initiate their transcription [3]. Both murine and human adipocytes exhibit extensive functional changes in culture in response to HIF-1, which alters the expression of up to 1300 genes [59]. These include genes encoding key adipokines, such as leptin, apelin, visfatin, TNF-α, IL-1, IL-6, VEGF, angiopoietin-like protein (Angptl)-4, MIF, PAI-1, and matrix metalloproteinases 2 and 9 (MMP-2, MMP-9), which are upregulated, and adiponectin, peroxisome proliferator-activated receptor (PPAR)-γ which is downregulated [3, 20, 55, 60, 61].

Hypoxia alters genes encoding key proteins for metabolic processes: glucose uptake, glycolysis, oxidative metabolism, lipolysis, and lipogenesis. Glucose uptake into adipocytes is stimulated by hypoxia because the expression of GLUT transporters is upregulated [20, 55, 62]. A switch from aerobic to anaerobic metabolism in hypoxic adipocytes is sustained by the increased activity of some glycolytic enzymes (e.g., phosphofructokinase [63]) and a net lactate release. Many studies focused on hypoxia-induced derangements of lipid metabolism reporting an increased lipolysis rather than unchanged but reduced lipogenesis in hypoxic adipocytes [64–66].

It seems that various degrees of adipose tissue hypoxia have different metabolic effects, and it is supposed also that subcutaneous and visceral adipocytes respond differently to factors that mediate tissue hypoxia. A recent study demonstrated that hypercaloric diet induces more severe hypoxia in mesenteric adipose tissue of mice than in the subcutaneous one [67].

Another direct effect of hypoxia is induction of insulin resistance via the upregulation of certain adipokines, the impairment of insulin-signaling pathway being a key change for white adipocyte dysfunction in obese subjects [3, 4].

Adipose tissue is one of the most plastic entities of an organism in terms of growth in the childhood and even in the adulthood in normal and pathological conditions, responding rapidly and dynamically to nutrient excess or starvation. Nor normal or pathological tissue, therefore nor the adipose tissue, is able to grow, develop, and function in the absence of an appropriate vascular network. Therefore, the hypoxia-induced expression of VEGF, the main angiogenic factor, and of certain adipokines, such as angiopoietin-2, Angptl-4, and leptin, sustains the stimulation of angiogenesis in obese adipose tissue [68–70]. Experimental data emphasize the induction of a pro-fibrotic switch of the transcriptional program in hypoxic adipocytes, fibrosis being another feature of adipose tissue dysfunction in obesity [29, 71]. Preadipocytes, pro-inflammatory cells, and fibroblasts from WAT as well as adipocytes respond to hypoxic conditions, favoring cellular events that lead to inflammation and fibrosis. Biostatistical analysis of WAT transcriptome had demonstrated a positive correlation between fat mass, degree of inflammation, and synthesis of ECM in obesity complications [72].

4. WAT hypoxia: a link between obesity and inflammation

The necessary link between abdominal (visceral or central) obesity and the development of type 2 diabetes and metabolic syndrome (which includes atherosclerosis, hypertension, and hyperlipidemia) due to the expanding fat mass and adipose tissue dysfunction was first demonstrated by Spiegelman's group [73, 74]. The mild inflammation status of the adipose tissue in obese subjects is induced by the peculiar role occupied by TNF-α, a 26 kDa transmembrane protein secreted as a cytokine and acting as an endotoxin-induced factor causing necrosis of tumors in vitro and cachexia in vivo, so naturally linked to the energy homeostasis [1]. They discovered that TNF-α is an active biofactor secreted by adipocytes and stromovascular cells positively correlated with obesity and insulin resistance.

Many signaling pathways have been proposed to be involved in the pathogenesis of obesity-associated inflammation called also "metaflammation" [75] such as (i) activation of toll-like receptor 4 (TLR4) by free fatty acids released after lipolysis [76], (ii) activation of protein kinase C (PKC) by diacylglicerol and ceramide [77]), (iii) induction of ER stress [25, 78] and oxidative stress [79], and (iv) adipocyte death [39]. Recent research data suggest that adipose tissue hypoxia is one of the first pathophysiological changes and was placed as a missing link between obesity and low-grade inflammation [61, 80].

Clinical and physiological data argue that in the whole organism the oxygen level is not the same in all the tissues nor constant for the same tissue and an isolate organ or tissue may lack oxygen even if the total supply is not compromised. This seems to be the case of the hypoxia inside the WAT human depots, the expanding adipose lobules or hypertrophic adipocytes resting isolated in pockets of tissue that lack the vascular supply, while other areas could be in normoxia or even hyperoxia [20]. The lack of oxygen perfusion for the hypertrophic adipocytes made them necrotic and finally they died. Dead adipocytes and free lipid droplets liberatedly act as recruitment factors for macrophages [39]. Besides adipocytes, preadipocytes and macrophages (the main players in WAT inflammatory response stimulating the inflammatory state in adipose tissue by the release of pro-inflammatory cytokines, such as TNF-α and interleukins) also respond to hypoxia. For such controversial results regarding the hypoxia in human adipose tissue, one must consider the technique accuracy and the methodological issues, minding that the same depot could be polarized toward hypoxic areas or inflamed and hypervascularized nests. Such a clustered differentiation is not unique in the adipose tissue since data demonstrated that in obese adipose tissue the switch from M2a macrophages discriminative for lean mice to M1 inflammatory phenotype takes place in well-defined spatiotemporal areas inside the same adipose depot [81].

In order to assess the involvement of TLR signaling in inflammation in obesity-related diseases, we analyzed the expression of TLR-2, TLR-4, TNF-α, and CD-68 in subcutaneous and visceral adipose depots from lean, obese, and obese diabetic subjects. We observed that both types of depots showed an increased number of small- and medium-dilated vessels with many CD68-positive cells [82]. In the peritoneal depots, we observed leukocyte margination with CD68-positive cells, but we didn't notice the presence of macrophages crowns in none of the samples analyzed, as Cinti and coworkers found in adipose tissue with hypertrophic cells [39]. Data obtained proved that same cells from the visceral adipose depots of obese and obese-diabetic patients, mainly macrophages, intravascular leukocytes, and endothelial cells, showed a positive reaction for both TLR-4 and TNF-α [82], proving that TLR4 activation contributes to the inflammatory process in obesity and the onset of the metabolic syndrome (**Figure 3**).

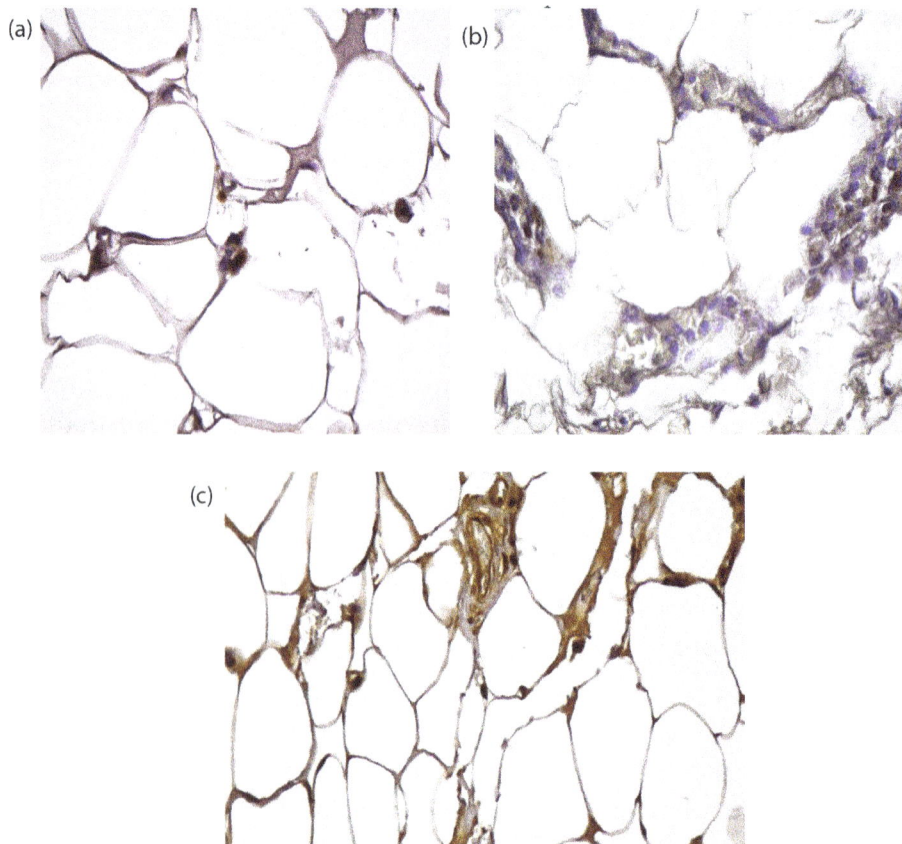

Figure 3. Immunostaining for CD68, TLR-4, and TNF-α of visceral obese adipose depots. (a) CD68-positive leukocytes between adipocytes (ob. ×40) in adipose peritoneal depots, (b) TLR-4-positive leukocytes and endothelial cells (ob. ×40), (c) intense-positive TNF-α reaction in visceral depots (ob. ×40).

Summarizing the data linking the cellular and molecular alterations of the adipose tissue in obesity to the adipose tissue dysfunction, among the three events highlighted—oxidative stress, ER stress, and local hypoxia—hypoxia might be the first in a logical chronologically order, since it promotes oxidative and ER stress. In obesity, quick changes from normoxia/ hyperoxia to hypoxia would be needed in order to induce oxidative stress [16]. Adipose tissue hypoxia induces inflammation through activation of two main transcription factors, HIF-1α and nuclear factor (NF)-KB, each of them activating transcription of a variety of genes encoding angiogenic and/or pro-inflammatory adipocytokines [26, 83]. Available data demonstrate that in rodent, HIF-1α upregulation starts in the first 1–3 days after the administration of a high-fat diet, before inflammation and insulin resistance develop [15, 19, 84].

5. Hypoxia: a major trigger for adipose tissue remodeling

Adipose tissue hypoxia is a concept that can practically explain the main alterations defining the adipose tissue dysfunction due to obesity: chronic inflammation, leptin expression, adiponectin reduction, adipocyte death followed by the invasion of monocytes and activation of macrophages, elevated lipolysis and adipocyte insulin resistance, and increased activity of ROS [3, 15, 55]. This entire cellular and molecular imbalance is followed by a compulsory adipose depot remodeling. The concept of remodeling of adipose tissue refers, as in all other entities, to the turnover of the cells and of the ECM in response to the requirement for growth and expansion of the adipose depots [85]. The molecules (cytokines, adipokines, growth factors, and proteases) involved in adipose tissue remodeling are synthesized and act as a permanent result of the cross talk between adipocytes and stromal cells.

5.1. Adipocyte death and inflammation

Adipocyte death is accepted as the main trigger for the adipose tissue remodeling [84], but the cause of this event is not consensual: the adipocyte size or the hypoxic milieu. In mice a positive robust correlation exists between adipocyte size and adipocyte death [39]. Consecutively macrophages are accumulating in crown-like structures being a source of numerous pro-inflammatory cytokines. A difference in the incidence of dead adipocytes was noted, the intra-abdominal cells being more susceptible than those of the inguinal depots. The clearance of the cellular detritus by the macrophages is the trigger for a homeostatic remodeling program that will allow the further expansion of the adipose depots that include matrix remodeling and vasculogenesis. Foci of adipocyte death are therefore areas where macrophages promote obesity-associated inflammation [39]. Interestingly, adipocyte loss is associated with phenotypic changes in stromal monocytic-macrophage cells. In a chronologically sequence, after the scavenging, the place occupied by the huge dead adipocytes was taken by small-size adipocytes, and the former hypertrophic adipose tissue became hyperplasic (Faust et al., 1984 cited by [84]). As a new study demonstrated that the macrophages are crowded in foci of hypoxic tissue, a second theory emphasizes that adipocyte death is caused by the hypoxia and the macrophages are trapped into the hypoxic areas by MIF [65, 86].

5.2. Hypoxia underpins adipose tissue fibrosis

There are several recent studies involving fibrosis of adipose depots in installing hypoxia and insulin resistance [27, 28, 87].

Scherer's research group proposed that in adipose obese tissues hypoxia is the most important driving force downstreaming the events associated with inflammation and fibrosis [27]. They found that in adipose tissue from the transgenic mice HIF-1α-ΔODD, in which a dominant-active deletion mutation of HIF-1α is overexpressed, fed with a hypercaloric diet, the transcription factor HIF-1α failed to promote the pro-angiogenic program by targeting genes, such as VEGF-A. Moreover, in these mice HIF-1α induces the fibrotic program by an increased synthesis of fibrotic proteins, such as lysyl oxidase (LOX), type I and type III collagens, tissue inhibitor of matrix metalloproteinases (TIMP)-1, and connective tissue growth factor (CTGF). Histology performed with trichromic staining revealed thick fibrotic streaks composed of type I collagen fibers, similar results being reported also for the adipose pads from obese human subjects [88].

LOX is a known target gene of HIF-1α, and in adipose tissue of ob/ob transgenic mouse, LOX is found in increased level compared to wild type [27]. LOX cross-links elastin and collagens in ECM and creates ECM-resistant bands of fibrosis. In adipose tissue of ob/ob mouse, these collagen bundle "streaks" are found outside the "crown-like" structures previously described [27, 39, 84]. The conclusion derived was that collagen synthesis and deposition could be anterior to the accumulation of macrophages surrounding the adipose cells because hypoxia-induced fibrotic program develops shortly after the high-fat diet is established [27]. So adipose tissue fibrosis is not necessarily induced by inflammation but could be rather an upstream phenomenon through the synthesis of HIF-1α and LOX.

From a different point of view, like in other tissues, adipose tissue fibrosis develops as a result of a persistent inflammation and a failure of the normal tissue repair with *restitutio ad integrum*.

Interestingly, fibrosis of adipose depots in obesity seems to display an otherwise intensity as the inflammation and hypoxia, those visceral seeming to be not only less fibrotic than those peripheral but also with a different distribution of collagen fibers, especially pericellular or intraparenchymatous [28]. As the visceral depots are more inflamed than the subcutaneous depots as we showed [88], this observation contradicts the accepted biological sequence that fibrosis develops as a result of an excessive and altered ECM synthesis and storage by resident cells activated in an inflammatory environment. This abnormal amount of fibrotic matrix in the subcutaneous adipose tissue could be explained if we keep in mind the histology of the host tissue where the adipose depots expand (the subcutaneous adipose tissue develops toward a much more dense tissue than the visceral one). In obese subjects fibrosis accumulates in pericellular areas—lining each adipose cell or a group of cells (interstitial fibrosis) and around the vessels (**Figure 4**).

Collagen phenotypes are also different, types I, III, and VI being present in pericellular position but only I and III form thick bundles appearing as interlobular septa surrounding more cells [28]. In visceral (omental) depots, the accumulation of fibers in pericellular position is associated with small adipocyte size and a lowest quantity of circulating triglycerides, proving that the subjects with smaller adipocytes have a less adverse metabolic profile [27, 89], so fibrosis may act as a protective reaction. In the adipose depots, the significance of type VI collagen seems to be peculiar, since its appearance changes dramatically through adipogenesis [90]. Transgenic mouse col 6KO ob/ob shows reduced necrotic cell death and consumes only a half of the amount of food that ob/ob strain [91] and type VI collagen levels correlate with hyperglycemia and insulin resistance [87, 92]. Obese humans expressed higher levels of type VI collagen and macrophage markers [92].

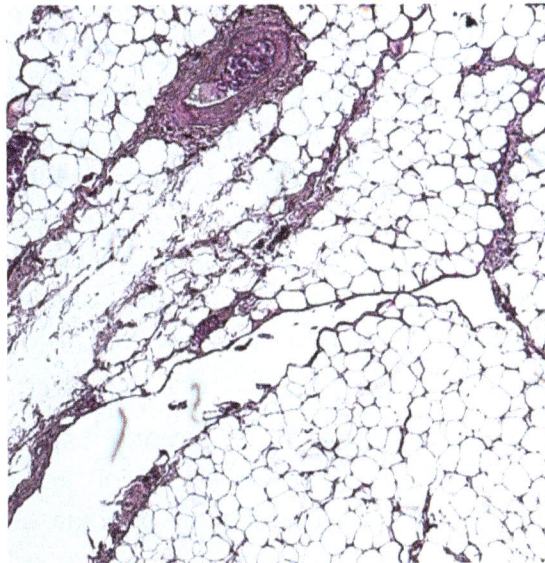

Figure 4. Pericellular and interstitial fibrosis in a visceral adipose depot from an adult obese subject (ob. ×20).

5.3. Hypoxia-induced angiogenesis in white adipose tissue

Being a compulsory condition for the expansion of any tissue, angiogenesis is a very limited process in normal adulthood (in endometrial cyclic physiology or wound healing), and the endothelial cells of the adult capillary network are in a relatively quiescent state.

In adipose tissue, angiogenesis is a very complex phenomenon regulated by a lot of molecules (hormones, cytokines, and growth factors) secreted by the stromo-vascular cells, including endothelial cells, and also by the adipocytes and preadipocytes [93, 94].

During adipose depot development, adipogenesis and vasculogenesis are temporally and spatially dependent, and in an adipose depot, the vascular network seems to act as a self-stop for the adipose expansion, since the inhibition of angiogenesis reduces the adipose tissue mass [95, 96].

In hypoxia induced by a high caloric intake, the vascular network does not progress uniformly between depots, due to the differences between the initial degree of vascularization and the rate/capacity of neovascularization during adipose tissue expansion. Hypoxia is more severe in mesenteric visceral depots than in subcutaneous [67], and at the same time, human visceral depots reveal a greater capillary density and angiogenic capacity than the subcutaneous adipose tissue [97, 98]. In their study using CD31+/CD34+ immunolabeling, Villaret and coworkers revealed that in obesity the capillary network is more developed and endothelial cell number is greater in visceral than in subcutaneous adipose depots, so increased hypoxia of visceral adipose tissue is not necessarily a consequence of capillary rarefaction [98]. The pro-angiogenic and pro-inflammatory phenotype of visceral adipose tissue could be related to endothelial cell senescence proved by an altered expression of some senescence markers such as IGFBP3, γH2AX, and SIRT1. They postulated at least two main causes for endothelial cell senescence in visceral adipose tissue: increased cell replication and oxidative stress [98]. Hyperplasia of obese visceral adipose tissue is responsible for an increased secretion of VEGF-A2 that stimulates endothelial cell proliferation.

The compensatory angiogenesis could prevent the metabolic disturbances induced by the hypoxia. It seems that not in all conditions the expansion of adipose tissue is associated with inflammation if an appropriate capillary bed is developed. If this condition is satisfied, the obese subjects are termed "metabolically healthy obese" because they may expand their adipocyte depots without inflammation consequences. This kind of expansion is associated with an enlargement of a given fat pad through recruitment of new adipocytes along with an adequate development of the vasculature, minimal associated fibrosis, and the lack of hypoxia and inflammation [83, 99].

The effects of hypoxia for obese humans have been recently disputed, the reactions triggered by the oxygen deprivation being a matter of severity, duration, and environment, since results between in vitro experiments, cell cultures under acute hypoxia, animal models, and human obese subjects are different. In recent studies, opposite data are reported by Goossens's research group. Their experiments revealed an increased pO$_2$ in obese insulin-resistant subjects and a positive correlation between pO$_2$ and gene expression for pro-inflammatory markers and an inverse association between pO$_2$ and peripheral insulin sensitivity [18]. In another experiment, after exposing mice at normoxia and hypoxia for the same duration of time, the authors reported a decrease in adipocyte size, macrophages infiltration, and inflammatory cell genes in adipose tissue from hypoxic animals [100]. The same results were reported for obese men exposed for 10 nights to hypoxia consecutively followed by increased insulin sensitivity [101]. Moreover, it was presumed that the obstructive sleep apnea could be a protective mechanism to maintain energy homeostasis in obese subjects [102, 103]. Angiogenesis in hypoxic tissues is controlled by HIF-1α, so-called the master regulatory of cellular and tissue response to hypoxic stress. In adipose hypoxic tissue, HIF-1 induces angiogenesis by upregulating VEGF gene. VEGF-A is the only endothelial growth factor that stimulates ECM degradation, proliferation, migration, and tube formation of endothelial cells [104]. VEGF secretion is regulated also by insulin stimulation, growth factor, and cytokines, such as PDGF, EGF, TNF-α, TGF-α, and IL-1β [99, 104].

As we showed in a previous study, VEGF immunohistochemical expression was higher in the adipose tissue of obese and obese-diabetic patients, especially in peritoneal depots. In normal weight subjects, both peripheral and central depots were VEGF negative [88].

It was demonstrated that an overexpression of VEGF in transgenic animals increased the vascularization and reversed the metabolic dysfunctions induced by a hypercaloric diet [80].

Recently, it had been claimed that the mechanism of VEGF promoting angiogenesis in adipose tissue is controlled by HIF-1β, while HIF-1α seems to regulate vascularization in BAT but not in WAT and additionally to promote WAT inflammation [105].

Adipokines, such as leptin and adiponectin, have also angiogenic properties that are stimulated in metabolically challenging conditions: leptin stimulates the angiogenic program upregulating VEGF expression, increases the vascular permeability by the formation of fenestrations in endothelial cells, and influences microvessel density [106]. For adiponectin, the results are conflicting: one supposed to be antiangiogenic because it inhibits endothelial cell migration and proliferation in vitro and neoangiogenesis in vivo [107] and others pro-angiogenic [99, 108].

6. Hypoxia: a trigger for BAT whitening and WAT browning

BAT presence has been reported once for small rodents and newborns, but recently, evidence for metabolically active BAT in adult humans has been reported [109]. BAT activation under β-adrenergic signaling is important for heat generation through uncoupled oxidative phosphorylation as a result of activation of non-shivering thermogenesis [110]. For this function, an important blood supply is required to provide the amount of oxygen and nutrients, and therefore BAT is much more vascularized than WAT. In relation to energy balance, an inverse relationship is accepted between BMI and age, BAT being less active in older subjects and in obese [111, 112]. Recent experiments highlighted the importance of hypoxia in BAT dysfunction too, the lack of an adequate BAT vascularization being involved in the overall dysfunction of the adipose organ in obesity [20]. BAT activity reduces the development of metabolic syndrome, and its activation increases insulin sensitivity and contributes to glucose homeostasis [113]. Having a high oxidative capacity, it is presumed that BAT is a contributor to systemic metabolic homeostasis, and this function was impaired in obesity, as demonstrated in the experiment performed by Shimizu and coworkers [114]. They proved in mice that obesity affects the density of the capillary network in BAT much more than in WAT and induced hypoxia in this organ. This elegant experiment shows in a very credible manner that the transition of phenotype from brown to white adipocytes is induced by the diminution of vascularization, a reverse mechanism of BAT differentiation observed in fetal development when the appearance of multilocularity is anticipated by the branching of the capillary loops (personal unpublished data). This vascular dysfunction is followed by the "whitening of the brown fat" (diminished β-adrenergic signaling, the appearance of enlarged lipid droplets in the cells and loss of mitochondria) and can impact obesity and obesity-related diseases [115]. HIF-1α increased level and suppression of UCP1 gene were observed in hypoxic BAT [114]. The same influences that hypoxia exerts on gene expression in WAT have been reported also for BAT, such as increased expression of leptin, VEGF, IL-6, and GLUT1. Due to loss of mitochondria, high glucose uptake will be accompanied by the same switch to anaerobic glycolysis as in WAT. Besides triggering inflammation in macrophages, lactate is supposed to be involved also in "browning of the white fat," recent experimental data proving that in vitro lactate induces the expression of genes encoding UCP1 and proteins involved in mitochondrial oxidation in mice and human white adipocytes [116]. Same authors demonstrated that lactate also controls the browning process in vivo because it regulates Ucp1 expression in a PPAR-δ-dependent manner, the combination of lactate and PPAR-δ ligand rosiglitazone constituting a strong inducer of an increased expression of some mitochondrial oxidation markers in mice white adipose depots [116]. Based on this observation, one can assume that lactate could be responsible for the recruitment of "brite" cells. In light of these results, the recruitment and activation of BAT are regarded as a potential new target for strategies to counteract obesity-induced changes.

In conclusion, hypoxia could be regarded as the leading cause of adipose tissue remodeling rather than as a consequence of the functional changes in the adipose organ. Due to the interplay between hypoxia, inflammation, and angiogenesis, targeting hypoxia pathways could be a valuable therapeutic approach to reduce the clinical consequences of the metabolic syndrome.

Author details

Ana Marina Andrei, Anca Berbecaru-Iovan, Felix Rareş Ioan Din-Anghel, Camelia Elena Stănciulescu, Sorin Berbecaru-Iovan, Ileana Monica Baniţă* and Cătălina Gabriela Pisoschi

*Address all correspondence to: monica.banita@yahoo.com

University of Medicine and Pharmacy of Craiova, Craiova, Dolj County, Romania

References

[1] Kershaw EE, Flier JS: Adipose Tissue as an Endocrine Organ. J Clin Endocrinol Metab. 2004;89(6):2548–2556. DOI:10.1210/jc.2004-0395

[2] Trayhurn P: Endocrine and signalling role of adipose tissue: new perspectives on fat. Acta Physiol Scand. 2005;184:285-293. DOI: 10.1111/j.1365-201X.2005.01468.x

[3] Trayhurn P, Wang B, Wood IS: Hypoxia and the endocrine and signalling role o white adipose tissue. Arch Physiol Biochem. 2008;114(4):267-276. DOI: 10.1080/13813450802 306602

[4] Trayhurn P: Hypoxia and adipose tissue function and dysfunction in obesity. Physiol Rev. 2013;93(1):1-21. DOI: 10.1152/physrev.00017.2012

[5] Berg AH, Scherer PE: Adipose tissue, inflammation, and cardiovascular disease. Circ Res 2005;96:939-949. DOI: 10.1161/01.RES.0000163635.62927.34

[6] McGee DL. Diverse Populations Collaboration: body mass index and mortality: a meta-analysis based on person-level data from twenty-six observational studies. Ann Epidemiol. 2005;15(2):87-97. DOI:10.1016/j.annepidem.2004.05.012

[7] http://www.who.int/mediacentre/factsheets/fs311/en/

[8] Kissebah AH, Vydelingum N, Murray R, Evans DJ, Hartz AJ, Kalkhoff RK, Adams PW: Relation of body fat distribution to metabolic complications of obesity. J Clin Endocrinol Metab. 1982;54(2):254-260. DOI:10.1210/jcem-54-2-254

[9] Carey VJ, Walters EE, Colditz GA, Solomon CG, Willet WC, Rosner BA, Speizer FE, Manson AE: Body fat distribution and risk of non-insulin-dependent diabetes mellitus in women, The Nurses' Health Study. Am J Epidemiol. 1997;145(7):614-619.

[10] Eckel RH: Obesity. Circulation. 2005;111(15):e257-259. DOI: 10.1161/01.CIR. 0000163653.38992.E5

[11] Gesta S, Tseng YH, Kahn CR: Developmental origin of fat: tracking obesity to its source. Cell. 2007;131(2):242-256. DOI:10.1016/j.cell.2007.10.004

[12] Janssen I, Katzmarzyk PT, Ross R: Body mass index, waist circumference, and health risk: evidence in support of current National Institutes of Health guidelines. Arch Intern Med. 2002;162(18):2074-2079.

[13] Khandekar MJ, Cohen P, Spiegelman BM: Molecular mechanisms of cancer development in obesity. Nat Rev Cancer. 2011;11(12):886-895. DOI: 10.1038/nrc3174

[14] Pasarica M, Sereda OR, Redman LM, Albarado DC, Hymel DT, Roan LE, Rood JC, Burk DH, Smith SR: Reduced adipose tissue oxygenation in human obesity: evidence for rarefaction, macrophage chemotaxis, and inflammation without an angiogenic response. Diabetes. 2009;58:718–725. DOI:10.2337/db08-1098

[15] Hossogai N, Fukuhara A, Oshima K, Miyata Y, Tanaka S, Segawa K, Furukawa S, Tochino Y, Komuro R, Matsuda M, Shimomura I: Adipose tissue hypoxia in obesity and its impact on adipocytokine dysregulation. Diabetes. 2007;56:901-911. DOI:10.2337/db06-0911

[16] Netzer N, Gatterer H, Faulhaber M, Burtscher M, Pramsohler S, Pesta D: Hypoxia, oxidative stress and fat, Biomolecules. 2015;5(2):1143-1150. DOI:10.3390/biom5021143

[17] Karpe F, Fielding BA, Ilic V, Macdonald IA, Summers LK, Frayn KN: Impaired postprandial adipose tissue blood flow response is related to aspects of insulin sensitivity. Diabetes. 2002; 51:2467–2473. DOI:10.2337/diabetes.51.8.2467

[18] Goossens GH, Bizzarri A, Venteclef N, Essers Y, Cleutjens JP, Konings E, Jocken JWE, Čajlaković M, Ribitsch V, Clément K, Blaak EE: Increased adipose tissue oxygen tension in obese compared with lean men is accompanied by insulin resistance, impaired adipose tissue capillarization, and inflammation. Circulation. 2011;124:67–76. DOI: 10.1161/CIRCULATIONAHA.111.027813

[19] O'Rourke RW, Metcalf MD, White AE, Madala A, Winters BR, Maizlin II, Jobe BA, Roberts CT Jr, Slifka MK, Marks DL: Depot-specific differences in inflammatory mediators and a role for NK cells and IFN-gamma in inflammation in human adipose tissue. Int J Obes (Lond). 2009;33(9):978-990. DOI: 10.1038/ijo.2009.133

[20] Trayhurn P, Alomar SY: Oxygen deprivation and the cellular response to hypoxia in adipocytes—perspectives on white and brown adipose tissues in obesity. Front Endocrinol (Lausanne). 2015;6:19. DOI: 10.3389/fendo.2015.00019.eCollection.2015

[21] Xue Y, Petrovic N, Cao R, Larsson O, Lim S, Chen S, Feldmann HM, Liang Z, Zhu Z, Nedergaard J, Cannon B, Cao Y: Hypoxia-independent angiogenesis in adipose tissues during cold acclimation. Cell Metab. 2009;9(1):99-109. DOI: 10.1016/j.cmet.2008.11.009

[22] Trayhurn P, Wood IS: Adipokines: inflammation and the pleiotropic role of white adipose tissue. Br J Nutr. 2004; 92(3):347-355

[23] Ye J, Gao Z, Yin J, He Q: Hypoxia is a potential risk factor for chronic inflammation and adiponectin reduction in adipose tissue of ob/ob and dietary obese mice. Am J Physiol Endocrinol Metab. 2007; 293(4):E1118-1128. DOI: 10.1152/ajpendo.00435.2007

[24] Wood IS, de Heredia FP, Wang B, Trayhurn P. Cellular hypoxia and adipose tissue dysfunction in obesity. Proc. Nutr. Soc. 2009; 68(4):370-377. DOI: 10.1017/S0029665109990206

[25] Koumenis C, Naczki C, Koritzinsky M, Rastani S, Diehl A, Sonenberg N, Koromilas A, Wouters BG: Regulation of protein synthesis by hypoxia via activation of the endo-plasmic reticulum kinase PERK and phosphorylation of the translation initiation factor eIF2alpha. Mol Cell Biol. 2002; 22:7405–7416

[26] Ye J, Gimble JM: Regulation of stem cell differentiation in adipose tissue by chronic inflammation. Clin Exp Pharmacol Physiol. 2011;38(12):872–878. DOI:10.1111/j.1440-1681.2011.05596.x

[27] Halberg N, Khan T, Trujillo ME, Wernstedt-Asterholm I, Attie AD, Sherwani S, Wang ZV, Landskroner-Eiger S, Dineen S, Magalang UJ, Brekken RA, Scherer PE: Hypoxia-inducible factor 1 alpha induces fibrosis and insulin resistance in white adipose tissue. Mol Cell Biol. 2009;29(16):4467-4483.

[28] Divoux A, Tordjman J, Lacasa D, Veyrie N, Hugol D, Aissat A, Basdevant A, Guerre-Millo M, Poitou C, Zucker JD, Bedossa P, Clement K: Fibrosis in human adipose tissue: composition, distribution, and link with lipid metabolism and fat mass loss. Diabetes. 2010; 59:2817-2825. DOI: 10.2337/db10-0585

[29] Reggio S, Pellegrinelli V, Clement K, Tordjman J: Fibrosis as a cause or a consequence of white adipose tissue inflammation in obesity. Curr Obes Rep. 2013;2:1-9. DOI: 10.1007/s13679-012-0037-4

[30] Kunduzova O, Alet N, Delesque-Touchard N, Millet L, Castan-Laurell I, Muller C, Dray C, Schaeffer P, Herault JP, Savi P, Bono F, Valet P. Apelin/APJ signaling system: a

potential link between adipose tissue and endothelial angiogenic processes. FASEB J. 2008; 22(12):4146-53. DOI: 10.1096/fj.07-104018

[31] Hajer GR, van Haeften TW, Visseren FLJ. Adipose tissue dysfunction in obesity, diabetes and vascular diseases. Eur Heart J. 2008;29(24):2959-2971. DOI: 10.1093/eurheartj/ehn387

[32] Cao Y. Adipose tissue angiogenesis as a therapeutic target for obesity and metabolic diseases. Nat Rev Drug Discov. 2010;9(2):107-15. DOI: 10.1038/nrd3055

[33] Cinti S: The adipose organ: morphological perspectives of adipose tissues. Proc Nutr Soc. 2001;60(3):319-328

[34] Cinti S: Adipocyte differentiation and transdifferentiation: plasticity of the adipose organ. J Endocrinol Invest. 2002;25(10):823-835. DOI:10.1007/BF03344046

[35] Frontini A, Cinti S: Distribution and development of brown adipocytes in the murine and human adipose organ. Cell Metab. 2010; 11(4):253-256. DOI:10.1016/j.cmet.2010.03.004

[36] Petrovic N, Walden TB, Shabalina IG, Timmons JA, Cannon B, Nedergaard J: Chronic peroxisome proliferator-activated receptor gamma (PPARgamma) activation of epididymally derived white adipocyte cultures reveals a population of thermogenically competent, UCP1-containing adipocytes molecularly distinct from classic brown adipocytes. J Biol Chem. 2010;285(10):7153-7164. DOI: 10.1074/jbc.M109.053942

[37] Seale P: Transcriptional control of brown adipocyte development and thermogenesis. Int J Obes (Lond). 2010;34 Suppl 1:S17-22. DOI: 10.1038/ijo.2010.178

[38] Chechi K, Carpentier AC, Richard D: Understanding the brown adipocyte as a contributor to energy homeostasis. Trends Endocrinol Metab. 2013;24(8):408-420. DOI: 10.1016/j.tem.2013.04.002

[39] Cinti S, Mitchell G, Barbatelli G, Murano I, Ceresi E, Faloia E, Wang S, Fortier M, Greenberg AS, Obin MS: Adipocyte death defines macrophage localization and function in adipose tissue of obese mice and humans. J Lipid Res. 2005;46(11):2347-2355. DOI:10.1194/jlr.M500294-JLR200

[40] Zhang YY, Proenca R, Maffei M, Barone M, Leopold L, Friedman JM: Positional cloning of the mouse obese gene and its human homolog. Nature. 1994; 372:425-432. DOI: 10.1038/372425a0

[41] Kahn BB, Flier JS: Obesity and insulin resistance. J Clin Invest. 2000;106(4):473-481. DOI: 10.1172/JCI10842

[42] Hotamisligil GS: Inflammation and metabolic disorders. Nature. 2006; 444:860-867. DOI:10.1038/nature05485

[43] Rosen ED, Spiegelman BM: Adipocytes as regulators of energy balance and glucose homeostasis. Nature 2006, 444:847-853. DOI:10.1038/nature05483

[44] Antuna-Puente B, Feve B, Fellahi S, Bastard JP: Adipokines: the missing link between insulin resistance and obesity. Diabetes Metab. 2008;34(1):2-11. DOI: 10.1016/j.diabet. 2007.09.004

[45] Skurk T, Alberti-Huber C, Herder C, Hauner H: Relationship between adipocyte size and adipokine expression and secretion. J Clin Endocrinol Metab. 2007; 92:1023–1033. DOI: 10.1210/jc.2006-1055

[46] de Souza Batista CM, Yang RZ, Lee MJ, Glynn NM, Yu DZ, Pray J, Ndubuizu K, Patil S, Schwartz A, Kligman M, Fried SK, Gong DW, Shuldiner AR, Pollin TI, McLenithan JC: Omentin plasma level and gene expression are decreased in obesity. Diabetes. 2007;56:1655-1661. DOI: 10.2337/db06-1506

[47] Cao R, Brakenhielm E, Wahlestedt C, Thyberg J, Cao Y: Leptin induces vascular permeability and synergistically stimulates angiogenesis with FGF-2 and VEGF. Proc Natl Acad Sci USA. 2001;98(11):6390-6395. DOI:10.1073/pnas.101564798

[48] Gabrielsson BG, Johansson JM, Lonn M, Jernas M, Olbers T, Peltonen M, Larsson I, Lonn L, Sjostrom L, Carlsson LM: High expression of complement components in omental adipose tissue in obese men. Obes Res. 2003;11:699-708. DOI: 10.1038/ oby.2003.100

[49] Dusserre E, Moulin P, Vidal H: Differences in mRNA expression of the proteins secreted by the adipocytes in human subcutaneous and visceral adipose tissues. Biochim Biophys Acta. 2000;1500:88-96.

[50] Tanko LB, Bruun JM, Alexandersen P, Bagger YZ, Richelsen B, Christiansen C, Larsen PJ: Novel associations between bioavailable estradiol and adipokines in elderly women with different phenotypes of obesity: implications for atherogenesis. Circulation. 2004;110:2246-2252. DOI: 10.1161/01.CIR.0000144470.55149.E5

[51] Fontana L, Eagon JC, Trujillo ME, Scherer PE, Klein S: Visceral fat adipokine secretion is associated with systemic inflammation in obese humans. Diabetes. 2007;56:1010-1013. DOI: 10.2337/db06-1656

[52] Blüher M: Adipose tissue dysfunction contributes to obesity related metabolic diseases. Best Pract Res Clin Endocrinol Metab. 2013;27:163-177. DOI:10.1016/j.beem.2013.02.005

[53] Hodson L, Humphreys SM, Karpe F, Frayn KN: Metabolic signatures of human adipose tissue hypoxia in obesity. Diabetes. 2013;62(5):1417-1425. DOI:10.2337/db12-1032

[54] Zhang L, Ebenezer PJ, Dasuri K, Fernandez-Kim SO, Francis J, Mariappan N, Gao Z, Ye J, Bruce-Keller AJ, Keller JN: Aging is associated with hypoxia and oxidative stress in adipose tissue: Implications for adipose function. Am J Physiol Endocrinol Metab. 2011;301(4):E599-607. DOI: 10.1152/ajpendo.00059.2011

[55] Ye J: Emerging role of adipose tissue hypoxia in obesity and insulin resistance. Int J Obes (Lond). 2009;33(1): 54–66. DOI:10.1038/ijo.2008.229

[56] Chen B, Lam KS, Wang Y, Wu D, Lam MC, Shen J, Wong L, Hoo RL, Zhang J, Xu A: Hypoxia dysregulates the production of adiponectin and plasminogen activator inhibitor-1 independent of reactive oxygen species in adipocytes. Biochem Biophys Res Commun. 2006;341(2):549-556. DOI: 10.1016/j.bbrc.2006.01.004

[57] Ambrosini G, Nath AK, Sierra-Honigmann MR, Flores-Riveros J: Transcriptional activation of the human leptin gene in response to hypoxia. Involvement of hypoxia-inducible factor 1. J Biol Chem. 2002;277:34601–34609. DOI: 10.1074/jbc.M205172200

[58] Blüher M, Wilson-Fritch L, Leszyk J, Laustsen PG, Corvera S, Kahn CR: Role of insulin action and cell size on protein expression patterns in adipocytes. J Biol Chem. 2004; 279:31902–1909. DOI: 10.1074/jbc.M404570200

[59] Mazzatti D, Lim FL, O'Hara A, Wood IS, Trayhurn P: A microarray analysis of the hypoxia-induced modulation of gene expression in human adipocytes. Arch Physiol Biochem. 2012;118:112-120. DOI:10.3109/13813455.2012.654611

[60] Rayalam S, Della-Fera MA, Krieg PA, Cox CM, Robins A, Baile CA: A putative role for apelin in the etiology of obesity. Biochem Biophys Res Commun. 2008;368(3):815-819. DOI:10.1016/j.bbrc.2008.02.2008

[61] Trayhurn P: Hypoxia and adipocyte physiology: Implications for adipose tissue dysfunction in obesity. Ann Rev Nutr. 2014;34:207-236. DOI: 10.1146/annurev-nutr-071812-161156

[62] Wood IS, Wang B, Lorente-Cebrian S, Trayhurn P: Hypoxia increases expression of selective facilitative glucose transporters (GLUT) and 2-deoxy-d-glucose uptake in human adipocytes. Biochem Biophys Res Commun. 2007;361:468-473. DOI: 10.016/j.bbrc.2007.07.032

[63] Rocha S: Gene regulation under low oxygen: holding your breath for transcription. Trends Biochem Sci. 2007;32:389-397. DOI:10.1016/j.tibs.2007.06.005

[64] De Glisezinski I, Crampes F, Harant I, Havlik P, Gardette B, Jammes Y, Souberbielle JC, Richalet JP, Riviere D: Decrease of subcutaneous adipose tissue lipolysis after exposure to hypoxia during a simulated ascent of Mt. Everest. Pflugers Arch. 1999;439:134-140.

[65] Yin J, Gao Z, He Q, Zhou D, Guo Z, Ye J: Role of hypoxia in obesity-induced disorders of glucose and lipid metabolism in adipose tissue. Am J Physiol Endocrinol Metab. 2009; 296:E333-E342. DOI: 10.1152/ajpendo.90760.2008

[66] O'Rourke RW, Meyer KA, Gaston G, White AE, Lumeng CN, Marks DL: Hexosamine biosynthesis is a possible mechanism underlying hypoxia's effects on lipid metabolism in human adipocytes. PLoS One.2013;8:e71165. DOI: 10.1371/journal.pone.0071165

[67] Michailidou Z, Turban S, Miller E, Zou X, Schrader J, Ratcliffe PJ, Hadoke PW, Walker BR, Iredale JP, Morton NM, Seckl JR: Increased angiogenesis protects against adipose hypoxia and fibrosis in metabolic disease-resistant 11β-hydroxysteroid dehydrogenase

type 1 (HSD1)-deficient mice. J Biol Chem. 2012;287(6):4188-4197. DOI: 10.1074/jbc.M111.259325.

[68] Bouloumié A, Drexler HCA, Lafontan M, Busse R: Leptin, the product of Ob gene, promotes angiogenesis. Circ Res. 1998; 83:1059-1066.

[69] Zhu H, Li J, Qin W, Yang Y, He X, Wan D, Gu J: Cloning of a novel gene, ANGPTL4 and the functional study in angiogenesis. Zhonghua Yi Xue Za Zhi. 2002;82:94-99.

[70] Ledoux S, Queguiner, Msika S, Calderari S, Rufat P, Gasc JM, Corvol P, Larger E: Angiogenesis associated with visceral and subcutaneous adipose tissue in severe human obesity. Diabetes. 2008;57:3247-3257. DOI:10.2237/db07-1812

[71] Sun K, Tordjman J, Clement K, Scherer PE: Fibrosis and adipose tissue dysfunction. Cell Metab. 2013;18:470-477. DOI:10.1016/j.cmet.2013.06.016

[72] Mutch DM, Tordjman J, Pelloux V, Hanczar B, Henegar C, Poitou C, Veyrie N, Zucker JD, Clément K: Needle and surgical biopsy techniques differentially affect adipose tissue gene expression profiles. Am J Clin Nutr. 2009;89:51-57. DOI: 10.3945/ajcn.2008.26802

[73] Hotamisligil GS, Shargill NS, Spiegelman BM: Adipose expression of tumor necrosis factor-alpha: direct role in obesity-linked insulin resistance. Science. 1993;259(5091):87-91.

[74] Hotamisligil GS, Arner P, Caro JF, Atkinson RL, Spiegelman BM: Increased adipose tissue expression of tumor necrosis factor-alpha in human obesity and insulin resistance. J Clin Invest. 1995;95(5):2409-2415. DOI:10.1172/JCI117936

[75] Gregor MF, Hotamisligil GS: Adipocyte stress: the endoplasmic reticulum and metabolic disease. J Lipid Res. 2007;48:1905-1914. DOI:10.1194/jlr.R700007-JLR200

[76] Shi H, Cave B, Inouye K, Bjørbaek C, Flier JS: Overexpression of suppressor of cytokine signaling 3 in adipose tissue causes local but not systemic insulin resistance. Diabetes. 2006;55(3):699-707.

[77] Yu C, Chen Y, Cline GW, Zhang D, Zong H, Wang Y, Bergeron R, Kim JK, Cushman SW, Cooney GJ, Atcheson B, White MF, Kraegen EW, Shulman GI: Mechanism by which fatty acids inhibit insulin activation of insulin receptor substrate-1 (IRS-1)-associated phosphatidylinositol 3-kinase activity in muscle. J Biol Chem. 2002;277(52):50230-50236. DOI:10.1074/jbc.M200958200

[78] Özcan U, Cao Q, Yilmaz E, Lee AW, Iwakoshi NN, Özdelen E, Tuncman G, Görgün C, Glimcher LH, Hotamisligil GS: Endoplasmic reticulum stress links obesity, insulin action, and type 2 diabetes. Science. 2004;306(5695):457-461. DOI:10.1126/science.1103160

[79] Houstis N, Rosen ED, Lander ES: Reactive oxygen species have a causal role in multiple forms of insulin resistance. Nature. 2006;440(7086):944-948. DOI:10.1038/nature04634

[80] Lefere S, Van Steenkiste C, Verhelst X, Van Vlierberghe H, Devisscher L, Geerts A: Hypoxia-regulated mechanisms in the pathogenesis of obesity and non-alcoholic fatty liver disease. Cell Mol Life Sci. 2016; April 18. DOI: 10.1007/s00018-016-2222-1

[81] Lumeng CN, DelProposto JB, Westcott DJ, Saltiel AR: Phenotypic switching of adipose tissue macrophages with obesity is generated by spatiotemporal differences in macrophage subtypes. Diabetes. 2008;57(12):3239-3246. DOI: 10.2337/db08-0872

[82] Fusaru AM, Stănciulescu CE, Surlin V, Taisescu C, Bold A, Pop OT, Baniţă IM, Crăiţoiu S, Pisoschi CG: Role of innate immune receptors TLR2 and TLR4 as mediators of the inflammatory reaction in human visceral adipose tissue. Rom J Morphol Embryol. 2012;53(3 Suppl):693-701.

[83] Sun K, Kusminski CM, Scherer PE: Adipose tissue remodeling and obesity. J Clin Invest. 2011;121(6):2094-2101. DOI: 10.1172/JCI45887

[84] Strissel KJ, Stancheva Z, Miyoshi H, Perfield JW, DeFuria J, Jick Z, Greenberg AS, Obin MS: Adipocyte death, adipose tissue remodeling, and obesity complications. Diabetes. 2007;56(12):2910-2918. DOI:10.2337/db07-0767

[85] Lee MJ, Wu Y, Fried SK: Adipose tissue remodeling in pathophysiology of obesity. Curr Opin Clin Nutr Metab Care. 2010;13(4):371–376. DOI: 10.1097/MCO.0b013e32833aabef

[86] Rausch ME, Weisberg S, Vardhana P, Tortoriello DV: Obesity in C57BL/6 J mice is characterized by adipose tissue hypoxia and cytotoxic T-cell infiltration. Int J Obes (Lond). 2008;32(3):451-463. DOI: 10.1038/sj.ijo.0803744

[87] Chun TH: Peri-adipocyte ECM remodeling in obesity and adipose tissue fibrosis. Adipocyte. 2012; 1(2): 89–95. DOI:10.4161/adip.19752

[88] Fusaru AM, Pisoschi CG, Bold A, Taisescu C, Stănescu R, Hîncu M, Crăiţoiu S, Baniţă IM: Hypoxia induced VEGF synthesis in visceral adipose depots of obese diabetic patients. Rom J Morphol Embryol. 2012;53(4):903-909.

[89] Hoffstedt J, Arner E, Wahrenberg H, Andersson DP, Qvisth V, Löfgren P, Rydén M, Thörne A, Wirén M, Palmér M, Thorell A, Toft E, Arner P. Regional impact of adipose tissue morphology on the metabolic profile in morbid obesity. Diabetologia. 2010;53(12):2496-2503. DOI: 10.1007/s00125-010-1889-3.

[90] Nakajima I, Muroya S, Tanabe R, Chikuni K: Extracellular matrix development during differentiation into adipocytes with a unique increase in type V and VI collagen. Biol Cell. 2002;94(3):197-203.

[91] Khan T, Muise ES, Iyengar P, Wang ZV, Chandalia M, Abate N, Zhang BB, Bonaldo P, Chua S, Scherer PE: Metabolic dysregulation and adipose tissue fibrosis: role of collagen VI. Mol Cell Biol. 2009;(6):1575-1591. DOI: 10.1128/MCB.01300-08

[92] Spencer M, Yao-Borengasser A, Unal R, Rasouli N, Gurley CM, Zhu B, Peterson CA, Kern PA: Adipose tissue macrophages in insulin-resistant subjects are associated with

collagen VI and fibrosis and demonstrate alternative activation. Am J Physiol Endocrinol Metab. 2010;299(6):E1016-1027. DOI:10.1152/ajpendo.00329.2010

[93] Rehman J, Traktuev D, Li J, Merfeld-Clauss S, Temm-Grove CJ, Bovenkerk JE, Pell CL, Johnstone BH, Considine RV, March KL: Secretion of angiogenic and antiapoptotic factors by human adipose stromal cells. Circulation. 2004;109(10):1292-1298. DOI: 10.1161/01.CIR. 0000121425.42966.F1

[94] Halberg N, Wernstedt-Asterholm I, Scherer PE: The adipocyte as an endocrine cell. Endocrinol Metab Clin North Am. 2008;37(3):753-768, x-xi. DOI: 10.1016/j.ecl. 2008.07.002

[95] Rupnick MA, Panigrahy D, Zhang CY, Dallabrida SM, Lowell BB, Langer R, Folkman MJ: Adipose tissue mass can be regulated through the vasculature. Proc Natl Acad Sci USA. 2002;99(16):10730-10735. DOI:10.1073/pnas.162349799

[96] Bråkenhielm E, Cao R, Gao B, Angelin B, Cannon B, Parini P, Cao Y: Angiogenesis inhibitor, TNP-470, prevents diet-induced and genetic obesity in mice. Circ Res. 2004;94(12):1579-1588. DOI: 10.1161/01.RES.0000132745.76882.70

[97] Gealekman O, Burkart A, Chouinard M, Nicoloro SM, Straubhaar J, Corvera S: Enhanced angiogenesis in obesity and in response to PPAR gamma activators through adipocyte VEGF and ANGPTL4 production. Am J Physiol Endocrinol Metab. 2008;295(5):E1056-1064. DOI: 10.1152/ajpendo.90345.2008

[98] Villaret A, Galitzky J, Decaunes P, Estève D, Marques MA, Sengenès C, Chiotasso P, Tchkonia T, Lafontan M, Kirkland JL, Bouloumié A: Adipose tissue endothelial cells from obese human subjects: differences among depots in angiogenic, metabolic, and inflammatory gene expression and cellular senescence. Diabetes. 2010;59(11): 2755-2763. DOI:10.2337/db10-0398

[99] Sun K, Wernstedt Asterholm I, Kusminski CM, Bueno AC, Wang ZV, Pollard JW, Brekken RA, Scherer PE: Dichotomous effects of VEGF-A on adipose tissue dysfunction. Proc Natl Acad Sci USA. 2012;109(15):5874-5879. DOI:10.1073/pnas.1200447109

[100] van den Borst B, Schols AM, de Theije C, Boots AW, Kohler SE, Goossens GH, Gosker HR: Characterization of the inflammatory and metabolic profile of adipose tissue in a mouse model of chronic hypoxia. J Appl Physiol. 2013;114:1619–1628. DOI: 10.1152/ japplphysiol.00460.2012

[101] Lecoultre V, Peterson CM, Covington JD, Ebenezer PJ, Frost EA, Schwarz JM, Ravussin E: Ten nights of moderate hypoxia improves insulin sensitivity in obese humans. Diabetes Care. 2013;36:e197–198. DOI:10.2337/dc13-1350

[102] Ye J. Hypoxia in obesity - from bench to bedside. J Transl Med. 2012; 10(Suppl 2): A20. DOI: 10.1186/1479-5876-10-S2-A20

[103] Goossens GH, Blaak EE: Adipose tissue dysfunction and impaired metabolic health in human obesity: a matter of oxygen? Front Endocrinol. 2015;6:55. DOI:10.3389/fendo. 2015.00055

[104] Liekens S, De Clercq E, Neyts J: Angiogenesis: regulators and clinical applications. Biochem Pharmacol. 2001;61(3):253-270

[105] Zhang X, Lam KS, Ye H, Chung SK, Zhou M, Wang Y, Xu A: Adipose tissue-specific inhibition of hypoxia-inducible factor 1{alpha} induces obesity and glucose intolerance by impeding energy expenditure in mice. J Biol Chem. 2010;285(43):32869-32877. DOI: 10.1074/jbc.M110.135509

[106] Christiaens V, Lijnen HR: Angiogenesis and development of adipose tissue. Mol Cell Endocrinol. 2010;318(1-2):2-9. DOI: 10.1016/j.mce.2009.08.006

[107] Brakenhielm E, Veitonmaki N, Cao R, Kihara S, Matsuzawa Y, Zhivotovsky B, Funa-hashi T, Cao Y: Adiponectin-induced antiangiogenesis and antitumor activity involve caspase-mediated endothelial cell apoptosis. Proc Natl Acad Sci USA. 2004;101(8): 2476-2481

[108] Kobayashi H, Ouchi N, Kihara S, Walsh K, Kumada M, Abe Y, Funahashi T, Matsuzawa Y: Selective suppression of endothelial cell apoptosis by the high molecular weight form of adiponectin. Circ Res. 2004;94(4):e27-31

[109] Zingaretti MC, Crosta F, Vitali A, Guerrieri M, Frontini A, Cannon B, Nedergaard J, Cinti S: The presence of UCP1 demonstrates that metabolically active adipose tissue in the neck of adult humans truly represents brown adipose tissue. FASEB J. 2009;23(9): 3113-3120. DOI: 10.1096/fj.09-133546

[110] Cannon B, Nedergaard J: Brown adipose tissue: function and physiological signifi-cance. Physiol Rev. 2004;84:277–359. DOI:10.1152/physrev.00015.2003

[111] Lee P, Greenfield JR, Ho KKY, Fulham MJ: A critical appraisal of the prevalence and metabolic significance of brown adipose tissue in adult humans. Am J Physiol Endo-crinol Metab. 2010;299:E601–606. DOI:10.1152/ajpendo.00298.2010

[112] Pfannenberg C, Werner MK, Ripkens S, Stef I, Deckert A, Schmadl M, Reimold M, Häring HU, Claussen CD, Stefan N: Impact of age on the relationships of brown adipose tissue with sex and adiposity in humans. Diabetes. 2010;59:1789–1793. DOI:10.2337/db10-0004

[113] Stanford KI, Middelbeek RJ, Townsend KL, An D, Nygaard EB, Hitchcox KM, Markan KR, Nakano K, Hirshman MF, Tseng YH, Goodyear LJ: Brown adipose tissue regulates glucose homeostasis and insulin sensitivity. J Clin Invest. 2013;123:215–223. DOI: 10.1172/JCI62308

[114] Shimizu I, Aprahamian T, Kikuchi R, Shimizu A, Papanicolaou KN, MacLauchlan S, Maruyama S, Walsh K: Vascular rarefaction mediates whitening of brown fat in obesity. J Clin Invest. 2014;124:2099–2112. DOI:10.1172/JCI71643

[115] Shimizu I, Walsh K: The whitening of brown fat and its implications for weight management in obesity. Curr Obes Rep.2015 ;4:224-228. DOI:10.1007/s13679-015-0157-8

[116] Carrière A, Jeanson Y, Berger-Müller S, André M, Chenouard V, Arnaud E, Barreau C, Walther R, Galinier A, Wdziekonski B, Villageois P, Louche K, Collas P, Moro C, Dani C, Villarroya F, Casteilla L: Browning of white adipose cells by intermediate metabolites: an adaptive mechanism to alleviate redox pressure. Diabetes. 2014 ;63:3253–3265. DOI:10.2337/db13-1885

Hypoxia-Induced Molecular and Cellular Changes in the Congenitally Diseased Heart: Mechanisms and Strategies of Intervention

Dominga Iacobazzi, Massimo Caputo and

Mohamed T Ghorbel

Abstract

Tissue hypoxia plays a critical role in the pathobiology of congenital heart diseases, especially with regard to cyanotic patients. Here, we describe the cellular and molecular mechanisms induced by hypoxia in the diseased heart, with particular attention to the metabolic and functional changes that underlie the hypoxia-induced right ventricle remodelling. The role of reactive oxygen species in transcriptomic changes, DNA damage, contractile dysfunction and extracellular matrix remodelling will be addressed. Furthermore, the reoxygenation injury, which occurs when oxygen is reintroduced upon initiation of cardiopulmonary bypass, will be discussed. This allows a better understanding of the risks associated with the reoxygenation injury in children undergoing open-heart surgery and helps to improve strategies of intervention for myocardial protection.

Keywords: hypoxia, congenital heart disease, cyanosis, reoxygenation injury, cardiovascular disease

1. Hypoxia in cardiovascular disease and congenital heart disease

The term hypoxia refers to a condition where the tissues are not adequately oxygenated, usually due to interrupted coronary blood flow or a reduction in arterial blood oxygen partial pressure [1]. With the heart being a highly oxidative organ, relying on high oxygen consumption for the work of its contractile machinery, it appears obvious that cardiac cells are very sensitive to oxygen deprivation [2]. Heart hypoxia, which originates as a result of disproportion between the amount of oxygen supplied to the cardiac cell and the amount required by the cell, plays a critical role in the pathobiology of several cardiovascular diseases [3]. These include myocardial infarction, coronary artery diseases, heart failure secondary to pulmonary disease and congenital heart diseases [1, 4, 5]. In patients with coronary artery diseases and myocardial infarction, hypoxia is usually due to the formation of an atherosclerotic plaque in the wall of coronary arteries, which reduces the perfusion of myocardial tissue [6]. In addition, a rupture of the plaque might result in complete arterial occlusion, leading to the death of the ischemic tissue [6]. The increased O_2 consumption caused by pressure overload and reduced O_2 delivery, due to impaired coronary blood flow, are the main causes of hypoxia in patients suffering from heart failure secondary to pulmonary hypertension [7].

The scenario looks different when shifting the focus to myocardial hypoxia in paediatric patients with congenital heart diseases (CHDs). Diseases affecting the heart, in fact, have usually a different pathophysiology in children compared to adult population [8]. Furthermore, as a result of the different pathophysiological function of the defective heart, the paediatric and adult patients are differently susceptible to stress insults, although there is still disagreement on whether the vulnerability of immature heart is less or more than for adult heart [9–12].

Congenital heart diseases include a wide spectrum of anomalies of the cardiac architecture, and they are usually classified based on the anatomical and pathophysiological nature of the defect. The main anomalies involve atrioventricular junctions and valves [i.e. atrial septal defect (ASD), ventricular septal defect (VSD), atrioventricular septal defect (AVSD)], the ventricular outflow tracts [like in tetralogy of Fallot (TOF)] or can consist of univentricular hearts [like single ventricle (SV)] [13].

More often, congenital heart defects are simply classified as cyanotic and acyanotic, depending on whether or not the defect affects the amount of oxygen in the body. In cyanotic heart defects, as consequence of a mixture between oxygenated and de-oxygenated blood, less oxygen-rich blood reaches the different tissues of the body, resulting in a bluish skin, lips and nail bed colour. This category includes defects such as TOF, transposition of the great vessels or truncus arteriosus. On the other hand, non-cyanotic CHD patients do not experience a lack in blood oxygen supply; therefore, they rarely develop the bluish colour, except for few occasion, when the baby needs more oxygen, such as when crying and feeding. Atrial and/or ventricular septal defects or coarctation of the aorta are examples of acyanotic CHDs [14, 15].

Several studies have shown that, among CHDs, cyanotic patients are much more prone to develop a severe chronic hypoxia state, compared to the acyanotic ones, as the lack of oxygen exposes the cardiac tissue to an increase in free oxygen radicals [16, 17]. Therefore, when considering the treatment of these patients, the oxidative stress problem has to be taken into account, in addition to the other anomalies that characterize these defects. Nevertheless, care must be taken also for the treatment of acyanotic patients, to prevent the hypoxia that might develop in a later stage.

2. Mechanism underlying the hypoxia response in Congenital Heart Disease

2.1. Depletion of antioxidant defences

The exposure of a defective heart to chronic hypoxia induces molecular and cellular changes that affect the myocardial function and metabolism. One of the most typical sign of a heart-developing chronic hypoxia is the unbalance between the level of reactive oxygen species (ROS) and the antioxidant defence system. ROS are physiologically produced during cell metabolic and energetic reactions [18]. Nevertheless, the body is endowed with antioxidant enzymes such as catalase, glutathione peroxidase, and superoxide dismutase and vitamins (retinoic acid, alpha-tocopherol, ascorbic acid) that can counteract this physiological production [19]. Even in case of excessive free radical production, the body responds to restore harmony balance [20]. However, under chronic hypoxia, a downregulation of antioxidant defences occurs, making the cells vulnerable to oxidant damage. Two different studies analysing the oxidant status of paediatric patients with CHDs revealed that the oxidative stress index, given by the ratio between pro-oxidants and antioxidants factors, was higher in the plasma of cyanotic children compared to the controls [16, 17]. No difference was found between acyanotic and control groups, thus confirming that the anatomical defect dictates the hypoxic level and the oxidative status [16, 17].

2.2. Hypoxia-induced metabolic and functional changes: the basis of right ventricle remodelling

Metabolic markers of oxidative stress, such as 8-isoprostane, were shown to be high in cyanotic patients' heart as revealed by our study evaluating the transcriptomic analysis of patients with tetralogy of Fallot (TOF) [21]. In a different study, we performed a genome-wide investigation to determine the global gene expression profiles associated with chronic hypoxia in the heart of patients with TOF, undergoing corrective cardiac surgery. The data revealed that 795 genes were differently expressed in cyanotic versus acyanotic hearts. In particular, genes associated with the contractility machinery function and MAPK signalling, involved in cell survival and antioxidant defence, were downregulated, whereas growth, remodelling and apoptosis-related genes were upregulated in the cyanotic group compared to the acyanotic one [22].

The altered gene expression triggered by the rise in reactive oxygen species is mostly responsible for the cellular and molecular changes that affect the myocardial function and metabolism, thus predisposing the heart to hypertrophy and failure. The hypoxia-induced downregulation of the sodium-calcium (Na^+–Ca^{2+}) exchanger (NCX1) in cyanotic patients decreases myocyte calcium handling capacity, leading to mechanical dysfunction [22]. In addition, ROS can induce oxidative modification of the sarcoplasmic membrane channels: the ryanodine receptor2 (RyR2) becomes abnormally activated while sarcoplasmic reticulum Ca^{2+}-ATPase (SERCA) is inhibited, causing an abnormal Ca^{2+} transient between cytosol and sarcoplasmic reticulum that contributes to the cardiomyocytes contractile dysfunction [23, 24]. ROS accumulation has also a detrimental effect on mitochondrial function by sustaining mitochondrial permeability transition pore (mPTP) opening and mitochondrial membrane depolarization. As a result, mitochondrial respiration is inhibited with less ATP production. The insufficient energy production also arises from the switch from an aerobic metabolism to a high glycolytic metabolic profile. Protein kinase D (PDK), which inhibits pyruvate dehydrogenase during glucose oxidation, is a key factor in the deficient energy supply [25, 26]. Another aspect of redox imbalance is the extracellular matrix (ECM) modification deriving from the matrix metalloproteinases (MMP) activation, which leads to heart remodelling and fibrosis [27].

Within the complex architecture of the heart, the right ventricle (RV) seems to be the most susceptible structure to be affected by the above-mentioned hypoxia-induced changes. The different morphology and metabolism between the left and the right ventricle can in part explain the different susceptibility [28]. Furthermore, the anatomy of most of the CHD exposes the right ventricle to higher stresses, making it more prone to fail than the left counterpart [24]. One of the main insults to which the RV is subjected is the pressure overload that can derive from pulmonary artery hypertension (PAH) or RV outflow obstruction, with both events leading to right ventricular hypertrophy (RVH) and eventually to right ventricular failure.

2.3. HIF-1alpha mediated angiogenic response

One of the key features of chronic hypoxia is the activation of the HIF-1alpha (HIF-1α) signalling, an essential regulator of the angiogenic response. The mechanisms by which HIF-1α is triggered are relatively well-understood: under hypoxia, HIF1-alpha degradation is prevented by the hydroxylation of specific protein residues, and therefore, its translocation to the nucleus promotes the transcriptions of pro-angiogenic genes like vascular endothelial growth factor (VEGF), platelet-derived endothelial cell growth factor/thymidine phosphorylase (PD-ECGF/TP) and erythropoietin (EPO) [29–31].

The role of HIF-1α in adult ischemic heart disease and pressure overload heart failure has been widely demonstrated by different research groups [6, 30, 32]. However, only few studies have investigated its involvement in the pathogenesis of congenital heart disease [6, 33, 34].

An important increase in HIF-1α and related pro-angiogenic genes and proteins have been reported in ventricular biopsies from children with cyanotic congenital heart disease, compared with acyanotic or control groups [22, 35]. In addition, mRNA level of HIF-1α as well as that of two of its representative target genes, VEGF and EPO, were found to be upregulated in blood samples of newborns with cyanosis and persistent pulmonary hypertension, therefore representing early markers of generalized hypoxia [36]. If the HIF-1α/VEGF-induced collateral vessel formation in hypoxemic myocardium is essential to compensate the lack of oxygen supply in cyanotic hearts, especially in cases of coarctation of aorta, an abnormal vessel formation can become a source of morbidity, due to arteriovenous malformations [34]. However, a correlation between VEGF increase and abnormal vessel formation has not yet been found [37]. Nevertheless, increased activation of HIF-1α/VEGF signalling might be detrimental in newborn with persistent pulmonary hypertension, as these patients normally present an overexpression of VEGF receptor 1 (VEGFR1), which accounts for the vasoconstrictor effect of VEGF [38].

Further mechanisms, independent from HIF-1α might account for the hypoxia-induced VEGF production in CHDs. As hypoxia is often associated with tissue damage and apoptosis, cytokines or other mediators (IL-10, TNF-α, TGF-β, etc.) might as well initiate the cascade that leads to VEGF production [31].

2.4. Hypoxia-induced DNA damage

The induction of p53 pathway, as a result of the ROS accumulation triggered by hypoxia, is one of the primary event that initiates the apoptotic cascade that occurs in hypoxic states. The activation of p53 leads to an altered expression of the pro-apoptotic gene Bcl-2, which, in turn, causes the DNA damage [39]. It has been shown that the extent of DNA damage depends on the anatomical anomaly and to the grade of cyanosis, with persistent cyanotic patients being more prone to DNA damage. In particular, children with TOF and with septal defects associated with great vessel anomaly displayed a significantly increased DNA damage compared to the ones with isolated septal defects [39, 40]. These data support the evidence that DNA damage can represent a marker of oxidative stress in CHDs as well as the common biochemical modifications and the oxidant status index.

2.5. miRNA involvement in myocardial adaptation to chronic hypoxia

Among the tissue and circulating biomarkers, microRNAs (miRNAs) have emerged as important tools to assess the hypoxic status of a variety of organs. Briefly, miRNAs are small (19–24 nucleotides) non-coding single-stranded RNAs that form complementary pair with specific target mRNAs to negatively regulate these mRNAs' expression via translational repression or degradation [41]. It has been documented that a hypoxic environment can alter the miRNA profile and their regulation of related pathways, especially with regard to apoptosis/proliferation functions [42]. Furthermore, intensive studies in cardiovascular field have shown how the heart pathophysiology is tightly regulated by miRNAs expression and function [43]. Several miRNAs (i.e. miR-208a, miR21, mi-R29) are involved in myocardial development, and their dysregulation has been linked to cardiac remodelling and hypertrophy; miR-145 upregulation was found in smooth muscle cells of vessels from both a murine model and patients with pulmonary arterial hypertension, whereas plasma upregulation of a huge number of miRNAs (miR-1, miR-133a, miT-499, miR-208) has been reported in patients with acute ischemia and, therefore, hypoxic myocardium [44–48]. Experimental studies performed on cardiac cells further validate the finding that miRNAs expression is modulated with hypoxic stimuli: 145 microRNAs were found to be differently expressed in a study conducted on the human cardiac cell cultured under hypoxia compared the normoxia [49]. Among these, miR-146b was shown to play an important role in the adaptation of cardiomyocytes to chronic hypoxia and its inhibition augmented hypoxia-induced cardiomyocyte apoptosis [50].

A wide array of miRNAs have been reported to be dysregulated in children with CHDs, most of which are crucial in RV development and are specifically linked to a particular defect [24]. In addition, the hypoxic state of some CHDs further affects the miRNA profile of the heart. A recent study by Huang and colleagues shed a light on miRNA-184 as a possible player involved in the mechanism leading to cyanotic CHDs [51]. miRNA-184 expression was, in fact, markedly decreased in myocardial samples from cyanotic CHDs patients, compared to controls and its suppression *in vitro* was also associated with decreased proliferation and induction of apoptosis, through a mechanism that likely involves the activation of Caspase-3 and -9 by the oxidised miRNA-184 [51]. In another study aimed to evaluate the involvement of miRNAs in the hypoxic response of cardiomyocytes, the expression of miR-138 in myocardial samples of cyanotic patients with TOF was almost twofold miR-138 expression in acyanotic group (VSD) patients [52]. This finding suggests that miR-138 might be used to discriminate TOF from other subtypes of CHDs and further supports the evidence that miRNAs can shed a light on the knowledge of the aetiology of different CHDs and be predictive of the clinical outcome/management of these diseases.

3. Reoxygenation and reperfusion injuries

After a hypoxic event or status of the heart, it is crucial to intervene to re-establish a normal oxygen level. In most cases, the intervention involves heart surgery with cardiopulmonary bypass (CPB) and cardioplegic arrest (CA). During such heart surgery, the standard protocol involves the administration of high level of oxygen upon initiation of CPB and before CA. This causes what is commonly referred to as reoxygenation injury [53]. Following the establishment of CPB, the heart is stopped (ischemic period) to carry out the corrective surgery. When the ischemic heart is reperfused at the end of intervention, a reperfusion injury occurs. The severity of this reperfusion injury depends on the severity of the ischemic period and may be linked to delayed post-operative recovery [54].

It has been widely reported that free oxygen radical formation plays an important role in the development of ischemia-reperfusion injury in the heart as well as in various organs. In the reperfused heart, this oxidant formation derives form a series of interacting pathways in cardiac myocytes and endothelial cells, which involve also leukocyte chemotaxis and inflammation. The white blood cells are, in fact, another great source of ROS: when activated by the binding to the hypoxic endothelium, they produce chemotactic substances and oxygen radicals, which are the main responsible for cellular damage [55]. In addition, nitric oxide (NO) production is greatly increased in post-ischemic hearts, thus impairing vascular reactivity [56].

It has been demonstrated that the damage resulting from the reperfusion event is more severe in hypoxic (low oxygen supply), compared to ischemic (low coronary flow) hearts [57]. When comparing the effects of reperfusion, respectively, in ischemic and hypoxic hearts, Samaja et al. found that the myocardial depression, the energy demand, and the associated O_2 free radicals were higher in the hypoxic rat hearts than the ischemic ones. Furthermore, the hearts subjected to chronic hypoxia are even more prone to the reoxygenation injury than the hearts that have experienced acute hypoxic events. The compensatory changes that occur in chronic lack of oxygen may account for the higher predisposition to generate larger amounts of oxygen radicals with the reintroduction of high levels of oxygen [58].

With many CHDs being characterized by a chronic hypoxic status, the subset of cyanotic children is obviously at a higher risk than the acyanotic CHDs population [59]. Clinical studies have shown that, despite similar cross-clamp times during open heart surgery, cyanotic children have worse clinical outcome and more reoxygenation injury, measured by troponin I release, compared with acyanotic children [11]. The major problem arises from the oxygen reintroduction during the cardiopulmonary bypass (CPB), which is a necessary procedure for the surgical management of CHDs [55]. As the chronic hypoxia produces long-term changes in the myocardial metabolism and function, the sudden oxygen reintroduction further exacerbates these effects. The impaired contractility due to hypoxia-induced calcium overload and the loss of high energy phosphates are examples of the pathological events amplified by the reoxygenation [59, 60]. In addition, the depletion of endogenous antioxidants that characterize chronic cyanosis cannot counteract the oxygen radical-mediated injury when oxygen is reintroduced [61]. On the contrary, minimal changes in the antioxidant reserve capacity were reported before and after the CPB in acyanotic infants, suggesting that, in the absence of hypoxia, a small amount of oxygen free radicals are produced [62].

The effect of reoxygenation injury due to CPB in corrective heart surgery in cyanotic children has further been proven by a significant change in the myocardial gene expression profile [21]. In particular, a wide genome expression array study found 32 significantly downregulated and three upregulated genes in cyanotic heart biopsies taken before and after hyperoxic CPB. Among the upregulated genes after reoxygenation, MOSC1, a factor involved in superoxide generation [63], showed a great increase at a mRNA level, thus suggesting its possible involvement in the increase in CPB-induced oxidative stress. On the other hand, the downregulation of the taurine transporter (TAUT) and the consequent depletion of the documented cardioprotective taurine [64] may in part explain some aspects of the myocardial injury, such as the mitochondrial and myofibers dysfunction. In addition, 8-isoprostane, a reliable marker of oxidative stress, was increased after CPB, and this correlated with the downregulation of keys genetic pathways related to myocardial function and to the reduction in antioxidant defenses [21]. It, therefore, appears obvious that the maintenance of endogenous antioxidants during hypoxia is a crucial determinant of tissue recovery on reoxygenation.

It has been suggested that HIF-α might as well stand as target for cardioprotection upon reoxygenation, by inhibiting mitochondrial oxidative metabolism and therefore reducing the generation of ROS under hypoxia-reoxygenation [6].

MicroRNA expression also appears to be affected by the reoxygenation event. In a study by Bolkier et al., the plasma levels of some cardiac-associated miRNA were dramatically increased after surgery of children undergoing open-heart surgery for CHDs. The increase in the selected miRNAs (microRNA-208a, -208b and -499) correlated with higher troponin levels and delayed hospital discharge [65]. This evidence further justifies the use of circulating miRNAs as biomarkers not only for the diagnosis but also for prognosis and prediction of surgical clinical outcome. In addition, through two different approaches—overexpression and inhibition—miRNAs might represent a suitable target to therapeutically treat those defect characterized by an altered expression of their level.

4. Strategies of surgical intervention

In order to reduce the risk associated with reoxygenation injury in children undergoing open-heart surgery, different interventional strategies have been explored. One of the strategies proposed to avoid this injury is the "controlled reoxygenation", achieved by using a partial pressure of oxygen in arterial blood (PaO_2) similar to the patient's preoperative oxygen saturation when starting CPB [66].

Before its adoption in current clinical practices, several experimental studies on animal models have provided the evidence that the biochemical and the functional status of the cyanotic heart are improved by delaying reoxygenation upon cardiopulmonary bypass. Morita and colleagues set up an *in vivo* experimental animal model where immature piglet hearts were subjected to hypoxemia followed by uncontrolled reoxygenation at high oxygen tension (400 mmHg) or controlled oxygenation at ambient tension (40 mmHg) followed by a raising in the tension to 100 mmHg first and 400 mmHg later. The authors found that lipid peroxidation was reduced while antioxidant reserve capacity preserved in the controlled-reoxygenation group, with this outcome correlating with improved ventricular contractility and functional recovery [67]. In addition, using a modified cold blood cardioplegia, enriched with potassium, the calcium influx was limited and the impaired contractility restored upon reoxygenation [66]. Similar results were obtained in another animal study where controlled normoxic reoxygenation showed a better outcome than abrupt oxygen reintroduction at high pressure. Furthermore, the effect of leukodepletion was examined in this study, in order to verify whether the removal of an important source of ROS, the white blood cells, would minimize the reoxygenation injury. The depletion of leukocytes from the blood-reduced oxygen free radical formation and preserved ventricular contractility at similar extent to the one achieved by controlled reoxygenation [55].

The beneficial effect of controlling the rate of re-introduction of molecular oxygen was also evident in adult patients. Lower lipid peroxidation and preserved antioxidant levels were observed in patients receiving normoxic reoxygenation, compared to the hyperoxic ones, although no significant difference between the two groups was found in the cardiac performance after CBP, likely because this was measured at one low time point of the Starling fraction curve [68]. The controlled-reoxygenation procedure has subsequently been adopted in the operations of cyanotic infants undergoing cardiac surgery, obtaining similar results to the ones seen in the acute experimental model [58].

Subsequent studies have further confirmed these findings and stressed the importance of controlled reoxygenation on starting CPB in cyanotic patients. In two randomized controlled trials including cyanotic children receiving CBP, we showed that the reduced myocardial injury in the controlled normoxic group was accompanied by a reduction in cerebral and hepatic injury, assessed by S100 and *α*GT measurement, which are markers of neuron and hepatocytes damage, respectively [69, 70]. In a different study, we have also analysed the effect of the two reoxygenation approaches on the myocardial gene expression profile of cyanotic paediatric patients undergoing corrective heart surgery. Results showed that the controlled reoxygenation reduced the transcriptomic alteration observed following hyper-oxic CPB. The most differentially expressed genes, mainly downregulated, were related to remodelling and metabolic processes, suggesting that the hearts subjected to hyperoxic reoxygenation had lower adaptation and remodelling capacity than the ones with controlled reoxygenation CBP [21].

Another approach of intervention, in the management of CPB, has involved the effect of whole body temperature during the paediatric cardiac surgery.

Although standard CPB procedures have always been conducted by cooling down the body temperature to 28° (hypothermic CPB), in order to reduce the metabolic rate and oxygen consumption, and therefore to protect organs from ischemic injury, recent evidences have demonstrated that normothermic (35°–37°) CPB is associated with lower inflammatory response and organ injury, both in adult and children [71–73].

In addition, we have shown that normothermic CPB in paediatric patients is also associated with reduced oxidative stress, assessed by troponin I and Isoprostane-8 release, compared with hypothermic CPB, while the inflammatory response has similar levels in the two groups [74].

Other researches have also investigated the effect of the temperature of cardioplegia during paediatric CPB. Warm blood cardioplegia, for long time adopted only in adult heart surgery, has proved to be safe and effective compared to standard cold CPB, with even better hydric balance and hemodynamic stability [75]. Once again, the pre-existent hypoxic status affects the biochemical and clinical outcome of the cardioplegic technique used. We have also shown that while for acyanotic patients the cardioplegic technique is not critical, for cyanotic patients, the use of cold blood cardioplegia with terminal warm blood cardioplegic reperfusion ("hot shot") improves the metabolic and functional recovery. The hot shot cardioplegia resulted in higher reperfusion ATP, ATP/ADP and glutamate levels than acyanotic patients, suggesting that this technique is advantageous only in stressed hearts [76]. Furthermore, the study shows that even if the blood cardioplegia is kept at cold temperature, this still offers a higher myocardial protection, compared to the crystalloid cardioplegia, confirming previous experimental and clinical results [77–79].

Besides CPB strategies, a pharmacological approach could be used as an interventional strategy for perioperative cardioprotection of hypoxic hearts. Experimental studies have shown that the selective inhibition of the enzyme phosphodiesterase-5 (PDE-5) can offer myocardial protection in infant hearts by improving myocardial function and reducing infarct size during reperfusion. However, no direct evidence between this protective effect and the hypoxia-induced injury was shown [80].

As for its established role in hypoxia, HIF-1α has also been investigated as a target for hypoxia-induced myocardial injury in reperfusion. By stabilizing its active form, through the compound dimethyloxyglycine (DMOG), a novel HIF-1α stabilizer, Zhang et al. showed that the progression of hypoxia-induced right ventricle remodelling was significantly reduced in a murine model of chronic hypoxia, most likely as a result of the induction of genes related to adaptive processes [81].

Furthermore, as previously mentioned, miRNAs are being extensively investigated as potential therapeutic tools in the management of CHDs. However, despite the fact that the road ahead looks promising and appealing, some obstacles, like the stability, the off-target effects and the immunogenicity of the delivery vehicles, still need to be overcome before getting miRNA-based therapeutics into clinical practice.

5. Conclusion

In conclusion, important steps ahead have been made in the knowledge of the mechanisms by which hypoxia takes part to the onset of congenital heart diseases, especially with regard to cyanotic patients. Likewise, significant advances have been made in the strategies of intervention involving open-heart surgery of children with these defects; in order to reduce the injury induced by CPB reoxygenation. Hopefully, the further understanding of the signalling pathways and the mechanism underlying the pathophysiology of hypoxia and hypoxia-induced reoxygenation injury in each kind of defect will result in the development of even better therapeutic strategies and in the design of specific interventions, particularly for the high-risk population.

Author details

Dominga Iacobazzi, Massimo Caputo and Mohamed T Ghorbel*

*Address all correspondence to: m.ghorbel@bristol.ac.uk

University of Bristol, School of Clinical Sciences, Bristol Heart Institute, Bristol, UK

References

[1] Essop MF. Cardiac metabolic adaptations in response to chronic hypoxia. J Physiol. 2007;584(Pt 3):715–26.

[2] Braunwald E. 50th anniversary historical article. Myocardial oxygen consumption: the quest for its determinants and some clinical fallout. J Am Coll Cardiol. 1999;34(5):1365–8.

[3] Ostadal B, Ostadalova I, Dhalla NS. Development of cardiac sensitivity to oxygen deficiency: comparative and ontogenetic aspects. Physiol Rev. 1999;79(3):635–59.

[4] Budev MM, Arroliga AC, Wiedemann HP, Matthay RA. Cor pulmonale: an overview. Semin Respir Crit Care Med. 2003;24(3):233–44.

[5] Grifka RG. Cyanotic congenital heart disease with increased pulmonary blood flow. Pediatr Clin North Am. 1999;46(2):405–25.

[6] Semenza GL. Hypoxia-inducible factor 1 and cardiovascular disease. Annu Rev Physiol. 2014;76:39–56.

[7] Shohet RV, Garcia JA. Keeping the engine primed: HIF factors as key regulators of cardiac metabolism and angiogenesis during ischemia. J Mol Med (Berl). 2007;85(12):1309–15.

[8]   Roche SL, Redington AN. The failing right ventricle in congenital heart disease. Can J Cardiol. 2013;29(7):768–78.

[9]   Starnes JW, Bowles DK, Seiler KS. Myocardial injury after hypoxia in immature, adult and aged rats. Aging (Milano). 1997;9(4):268–76.

[10] Jonas RA. Myocardial protection for neonates and infants. Thorac Cardiovasc Surg. 1998;46(Suppl. 2):288–91.

[11] Imura H, Caputo M, Parry A, Pawade A, Angelini GD, Suleiman MS. Age-dependent and hypoxia-related differences in myocardial protection during pediatric open heart surgery. Circulation. 2001;103(11):1551–6.

[12] Lopaschuk GD, Spafford MA. Differences in myocardial ischemic tolerance between 1- and 7-day-old rabbits. Can J Physiol Pharmacol. 1992;70(10):1315–23.

[13] Houyel L, Khoshnood B, Anderson RH, Lelong N, Thieulin AC, Goffinet F, et al. Population-based evaluation of a suggested anatomic and clinical classification of congenital heart defects based on the International Paediatric and Congenital Cardiac Code. Orphanet J Rare Dis. 2011;6:64.

[14] Fraser CD, Carberry KE. Congenital heart disease. In: Townsend CM Jr, Beauchamp RD, Evers BM, Mattox KL, eds. *Sabiston Textbook of Surgery*. 19th ed. Philadelphia, PA: Elsevier Saunders; 2012:chap 59.

[15] Webb GD, Smallhorn JF, Therrien J, Redington AN. Congenital heart disease. In: Mann DL, Zipes DP, Libby P, Bonow RO, *Braunwald E, eds. Braunwald's Heart Disease: A Textbook of Cardiovascular Medicine*. 10th ed. Philadelphia, PA: Elsevier Saunders; 2015:chap 62.

[16] Rokicki W, Strzalkowski A, Klapcinska B, Danch A, Sobczak A. Antioxidant status in newborns and infants suffering from congenital heart defects. Wiad Lek. 2003;56(7–8):337–40.

[17] Ercan S, Cakmak A, Kosecik M, Erel O. The oxidative state of children with cyanotic and acyanotic congenital heart disease. Anadolu Kardiyol Derg. 2009;9(6):486–90.

[18] Scandalios JG. The rise of ROS. Trends Biochem Sci. 2002;27(9):483–6.

[19] Birben E, Sahiner UM, Sackesen C, Erzurum S, Kalayci O. Oxidative stress and antioxidant defense. World Allergy Organ J. 2012;5(1):9–19.

[20] Espinosa-Diez C, Miguel V, Mennerich D, Kietzmann T, Sanchez-Perez P, Cadenas S, et al. Antioxidant responses and cellular adjustments to oxidative stress. Redox Biol. 2015;6:183–97.

[21] Ghorbel MT, Mokhtari A, Sheikh M, Angelini GD, Caputo M. Controlled reoxygenation cardiopulmonary bypass is associated with reduced transcriptomic changes in cyanotic tetralogy of Fallot patients undergoing surgery. Physiol Genomics. 2012;44(22):1098–106.

[22] Ghorbel MT, Cherif M, Jenkins E, Mokhtari A, Kenny D, Angelini GD, et al. Transcriptomic analysis of patients with tetralogy of Fallot reveals the effect of chronic hypoxia on myocardial gene expression. J Thorac Cardiovasc Surg. 2010;140(2):337–45.e26.

[23] Sharma K, Kass DA. Heart failure with preserved ejection fraction: mechanisms, clinical features, and therapies. Circ Res. 2014;115(1):79–96.

[24] Iacobazzi D, Suleiman MS, Ghorbel M, George SJ, Caputo M, Tulloh RM. Cellular and molecular basis of RV hypertrophy in congenital heart disease. Heart. 2016;102(1):12–7.

[25] Piao L, Sidhu VK, Fang YH, Ryan JJ, Parikh KS, Hong Z, et al. FOXO1-mediated upregulation of pyruvate dehydrogenase kinase-4 (PDK4) decreases glucose oxidation and impairs right ventricular function in pulmonary hypertension: therapeutic benefits of dichloroacetate. J Mol Med (Berl). 2013;91(3):333–46.

[26] Ryan JJ, Archer SL. The right ventricle in pulmonary arterial hypertension: disorders of metabolism, angiogenesis and adrenergic signaling in right ventricular failure. Circ Res. 2014;115(1):176–88.

[27] Qipshidze N, Tyagi N, Metreveli N, Lominadze D, Tyagi SC. Autophagy mechanism of right ventricular remodeling in murine model of pulmonary artery constriction. Am J Physiol Heart Circ Physiol. 2012;302(3):H688–96.

[28] Friedberg MK, Redington AN. Right versus left ventricular failure: differences, similarities, and interactions. Circulation. 2014;129(9):1033–44.

[29] Jaakkola P, Mole DR, Tian YM, Wilson MI, Gielbert J, Gaskell SJ, et al. Targeting of HIF-alpha to the von Hippel-Lindau ubiquitylation complex by O2-regulated prolyl hydroxylation. Science. 2001;292(5516):468–72.

[30] Semenza GL. O2-regulated gene expression: transcriptional control of cardiorespiratory physiology by HIF-1. J Appl Physiol (1985). 2004;96(3):1173–7; discussion 0-2.

[31] Felmeden DC, Blann AD, Lip GY. Angiogenesis: basic pathophysiology and implications for disease. Eur Heart J. 2003;24(7):586–603.

[32] Holscher M, Silter M, Krull S, von Ahlen M, Hesse A, Schwartz P, et al. Cardiomyocyte-specific prolyl-4-hydroxylase domain 2 knock out protects from acute myocardial ischemic injury. J Biol Chem. 2011;286(13):11185–94.

[33] Himeno W, Akagi T, Furui J, Maeno Y, Ishii M, Kosai K, et al. Increased angiogenic growth factor in cyanotic congenital heart disease. Pediatr Cardiol. 2003;24(2):127–32.

[34] El-Melegy NT, Mohamed NA. Angiogenic biomarkers in children with congenital heart disease: possible implications. Ital J Pediatr. 2010;36:32.

[35] Qing M, Gorlach A, Schumacher K, Woltje M, Vazquez-Jimenez JF, Hess J, et al. The hypoxia-inducible factor HIF-1 promotes intramyocardial expression of VEGF in infants with congenital cardiac defects. Basic Res Cardiol. 2007;102(3):224–32.

[36] Lemus-Varela ML, Flores-Soto ME, Cervantes-Munguia R, Torres-Mendoza BM, Gudino-Cabrera G, Chaparro-Huerta V, et al. Expression of HIF-1 alpha, VEGF and EPO in peripheral blood from patients with two cardiac abnormalities associated with hypoxia. Clin Biochem. 2010;43(3):234–9.

[37] Ootaki Y, Yamaguchi M, Yoshimura N, Oka S, Yoshida M, Hasegawa T. Vascular endothelial growth factor in children with congenital heart disease. Ann Thorac Surg. 2003;75(5):1523–6.

[38] Nadeau S, Baribeau J, Janvier A, Perreault T. Changes in expression of vascular endothelial growth factor and its receptors in neonatal hypoxia-induced pulmonary hypertension. Pediatr Res. 2005;58(2):199–205.

[39] Vidya G, Suma HY, Vishnu Bhat B, Parkash Chand, Ramachandra Rao K. Hypoxia induced DNA damage in children with isolated septal defect and septal defect with great vessel anomaly of heart. J Clin Diagn Res. 2014;8(4):SC01–3.

[40] Srujana K, Begum SS, Rao KN, Devi GS, Jyothy A, Prasad MH. Application of the comet assay for assessment of oxidative DNA damage in circulating lymphocytes of Tetralogy of Fallot patients. Mutat Res. 2010;688(1–2):62–5.

[41] Bartel DP. MicroRNAs: genomics, biogenesis, mechanism, and function. Cell. 2004;116(2):281–97.

[42] Kulshreshtha R, Ferracin M, Wojcik SE, Garzon R, Alder H, Agosto-Perez FJ, et al. A microRNA signature of hypoxia. Mol Cell Biol. 2007;27(5):1859–67.

[43] Condorelli G, Latronico MV, Cavarretta E. microRNAs in cardiovascular diseases: current knowledge and the road ahead. J Am Coll Cardiol. 2014;63(21):2177–87.

[44] Thum T, Gross C, Fiedler J, Fischer T, Kissler S, Bussen M, et al. MicroRNA-21 contributes to myocardial disease by stimulating MAP kinase signalling in fibroblasts. Nature. 2008;456(7224):980–4.

[45] van Rooij E, Sutherland LB, Thatcher JE, DiMaio JM, Naseem RH, Marshall WS, et al. Dysregulation of microRNAs after myocardial infarction reveals a role of miR-29 in cardiac fibrosis. Proc Natl Acad Sci U S A. 2008;105(35):13027–32.

[46] Caruso P, Dempsie Y, Stevens HC, McDonald RA, Long L, Lu R, et al. A role for miR-145 in pulmonary arterial hypertension: evidence from mouse models and patient samples. Circ Res. 2012;111(3):290–300.

[47] Wang GK, Zhu JQ, Zhang JT, Li Q, Li Y, He J, et al. Circulating microRNA: a novel potential biomarker for early diagnosis of acute myocardial infarction in humans. Eur Heart J. 2010;31(6):659–66.

[48] Cheng Y, Tan N, Yang J, Liu X, Cao X, He P, et al. A translational study of circulating cell-free microRNA-1 in acute myocardial infarction. Clin Sci (Lond). 2010;119(2):87–95.

[49] Chen YT, Liew OW, Richards AM. MicroRNA expression profiles of human left ventricle derived cardiac cells in normoxic and hypoxic conditions. Genom Data. 2015;5:59–60.

[50] Li JW, He SY, Feng ZZ, Zhao L, Jia WK, Liu P, et al. MicroRNA-146b inhibition augments hypoxia-induced cardiomyocyte apoptosis. Mol Med Rep. 2015;12(5):6903–10.

[51] Huang J, Li X, Li H, Su Z, Wang J, Zhang H. Down-regulation of microRNA-184 contributes to the development of cyanotic congenital heart diseases. Int J Clin Exp Pathol. 2015;8(11):14221–7.

[52] He S, Liu P, Jian Z, Li J, Zhu Y, Feng Z, et al. miR-138 protects cardiomyocytes from hypoxia-induced apoptosis via MLK3/JNK/c-jun pathway. Biochem Biophys Res Commun. 2013;441(4):763–9.

[53] Tan S, Yokoyama Y, Wang Z, Zhou F, Nielsen V, Murdoch AD, et al. Hypoxia-reoxygenation is as damaging as ischemia-reperfusion in the rat liver. Crit Care Med. 1998;26(6):1089–95.

[54] Ferrari R, Alfieri O, Curello S, Ceconi C, Cargnoni A, Marzollo P, et al. Occurrence of oxidative stress during reperfusion of the human heart. Circulation. 1990;81(1):201–11.

[55] Allen BS, Ilbawi MN. Hypoxia, reoxygenation and the role of systemic leukodepletion in pediatric heart surgery. Perfusion. 2001;16(Suppl):19–29.

[56] Zweier JL, Talukder MA. The role of oxidants and free radicals in reperfusion injury. Cardiovasc Res. 2006;70(2):181–90.

[57] Samaja M, Motterlini R, Santoro F, Dell' Antonio G, Corno A. Oxidative injury in reoxygenated and reperfused hearts. Free Radic Biol Med. 1994;16(2):255–62.

[58] Allen BS, Rahman S, Ilbawi MN, Kronon M, Bolling KS, Halldorsson AO, et al. Detrimental effects of cardiopulmonary bypass in cyanotic infants: preventing the reoxygenation injury. Ann Thorac Surg. 1997;64(5):1381–7; discussion 7-8.

[59] Corno AF, Milano G, Samaja M, Tozzi P, von Segesser LK. Chronic hypoxia: a model for cyanotic congenital heart defects. J Thorac Cardiovasc Surg. 2002;124(1):105–12.

[60] Najm HK, Wallen WJ, Belanger MP, Williams WG, Coles JG, Van Arsdell GS, et al. Does the degree of cyanosis affect myocardial adenosine triphosphate levels and function in children undergoing surgical procedures for congenital heart disease? J Thorac Cardiovasc Surg. 2000;119(3):515–24.

[61] Teoh KH, Mickle DA, Weisel RD, Li RK, Tumiati LC, Coles JG, et al. Effect of oxygen tension and cardiovascular operations on the myocardial antioxidant enzyme activities in patients with tetralogy of Fallot and aorta-coronary bypass. J Thorac Cardiovasc Surg. 1992;104(1):159–64.

[62] Bolling KS, Halldorsson A, Allen BS, Rahman S, Wang T, Kronon M, et al. Prevention of the hypoxic reoxygenation injury with the use of a leukocyte-depleting filter. J Thorac Cardiovasc Surg. 1997;113(6):1081–9; discussion 9-90.

[63] Morita K, Ihnken K, Buckberg GD, Sherman MP, Young HH. Studies of hypoxemic/reoxygenation injury: without aortic clamping. IX. Importance of avoiding perioperative hyperoxemia in the setting of previous cyanosis. J Thorac Cardiovasc Surg. 1995;110(4 Pt 2):1235–44.

[64] Ito T, Kimura Y, Uozumi Y, Takai M, Muraoka S, Matsuda T, et al. Taurine depletion caused by knocking out the taurine transporter gene leads to cardiomyopathy with cardiac atrophy. J Mol Cell Cardiol. 2008;44(5):927–37.

[65] Bolkier Y, Nevo-Caspi Y, Salem Y, Vardi A, Mishali D, Paret G. Micro-RNA-208a, -208b, and -499 as biomarkers for myocardial damage after cardiac surgery in children. Pediatr Crit Care Med. 2016;17(4):e193–7.

[66] Ihnken K, Morita K, Buckberg GD. Delayed cardioplegic reoxygenation reduces reoxygenation injury in cyanotic immature hearts. Ann Thorac Surg. 1998;66(1):177–82.

[67] Morita K, Ihnken K, Buckberg GD. Studies of hypoxemic/reoxygenation injury: with aortic clamping. XII. Delay of cardiac reoxygenation damage in the presence of cyanosis: a new concept of controlled cardiac reoxygenation. J Thorac Cardiovasc Surg. 1995;110(4 Pt 2):1265–73.

[68] Ihnken K, Winkler A, Schlensak C, Sarai K, Neidhart G, Unkelbach U, et al. Normoxic cardiopulmonary bypass reduces oxidative myocardial damage and nitric oxide during cardiac operations in the adult. J Thorac Cardiovasc Surg. 1998;116(2):327–34.

[69] Caputo M, Mokhtari A, Rogers CA, Panayiotou N, Chen Q, Ghorbel MT, et al. The effects of normoxic versus hyperoxic cardiopulmonary bypass on oxidative stress and inflammatory response in cyanotic pediatric patients undergoing open cardiac surgery: a randomized controlled trial. J Thorac Cardiovasc Surg. 2009;138(1):206–14.

[70] Caputo M, Mokhtari A, Miceli A, Ghorbel MT, Angelini GD, Parry AJ, et al. Controlled reoxygenation during cardiopulmonary bypass decreases markers of organ damage, inflammation, and oxidative stress in single-ventricle patients undergoing pediatric heart surgery. J Thorac Cardiovasc Surg. 2014;148(3):792–801, e8; discussion 0-1.

[71] Birdi I, Caputo M, Underwood M, Angelini GD, Bryan AJ. Influence of normothermic systemic perfusion temperature on cold myocardial protection during coronary artery bypass surgery. Cardiovasc Surg. 1999;7(3):369–74.

[72] Birdi I, Regragui I, Izzat MB, Bryan AJ, Angelini GD. Influence of normothermic systemic perfusion during coronary artery bypass operations: a randomized prospective study. J Thorac Cardiovasc Surg. 1997;114(3):475–81.

[73] Ohata T, Sawa Y, Kadoba K, Taniguchi K, Ichikawa H, Masai T, et al. Normothermia has beneficial effects in cardiopulmonary bypass attenuating inflammatory reactions. ASAIO J. 1995;41(3):M288–91.

[74] Caputo M, Bays S, Rogers CA, Pawade A, Parry AJ, Suleiman S, et al. Randomized comparison between normothermic and hypothermic cardiopulmonary bypass in pediatric open-heart surgery. Ann Thorac Surg. 2005;80(3):982–8.

[75] Durandy Y, Hulin S. Intermittent warm blood cardioplegia in the surgical treatment of congenital heart disease: clinical experience with 1400 cases. J Thorac Cardiovasc Surg. 2007;133(1):241–6.

[76] Modi P, Suleiman MS, Reeves B, Pawade A, Parry AJ, Angelini GD, et al. Myocardial metabolic changes during pediatric cardiac surgery: a randomized study of 3 cardioplegic techniques. J Thorac Cardiovasc Surg. 2004;128(1):67–75.

[77] Bolling K, Kronon M, Allen BS, Wang T, Ramon S, Feinberg H. Myocardial protection in normal and hypoxically stressed neonatal hearts: the superiority of blood versus crystalloid cardioplegia. J Thorac Cardiovasc Surg. 1997;113(6):994–1003; discussion 1003-5.

[78] del Nido PJ, Mickle DA, Wilson GJ, Benson LN, Weisel RD, Coles JG, et al. Inadequate myocardial protection with cold cardioplegic arrest during repair of tetralogy of Fallot. J Thorac Cardiovasc Surg. 1988;95(2):223–9.

[79] Modi P, Imura H, Caputo M, Pawade A, Parry A, Angelini GD, et al. Cardiopulmonary bypass-induced myocardial reoxygenation injury in pediatric patients with cyanosis. J Thorac Cardiovasc Surg. 2002;124(5):1035–6.

[80] Bremer YA, Salloum F, Ockaili R, Chou E, Moskowitz WB, Kukreja RC. Sildenafil citrate (viagra) induces cardioprotective effects after ischemia/reperfusion injury in infant rabbits. Pediatr Res. 2005;57(1):22–7.

[81] Zhang S, Ma K, Liu Y, Pan X, Chen Q, Qi L, et al. Stabilization of hypoxia-inducible factor by DMOG inhibits development of chronic hypoxia-induced right ventricular remodeling. J Cardiovasc Pharmacol. 2016;67(1):68–75.

3

Hypoxia and its Emerging Therapeutics in Neurodegenerative, Inflammatory and Renal Diseases

Deepak Bhatia, Mohammad Sanaei Ardekani,

Qiwen Shi and Shahrzad Movafagh

Abstract

Hypoxia is a common underlying condition of many disease states. Hypoxia can occur with ischemia, a lack of blood flow to tissues, or independent of ischemia as in acute lung injury, anemia, and carbon monoxide poisoning. Hypoxia may be observed in patients with diseases such as obstructive sleep apnea, cerebrovascular diseases, systemic hypertension, cardiovascular diseases, chronic obstructive pulmonary disease (COPD), pulmonary hypertension and congestive heart failure (CHF), inflammatory disease states, and acute and chronic renal diseases. In the past decade, research has shown hypoxic signaling to be involved in a range of responses from adaptation of the body to reduced oxygen to pathogenesis of disease. Hypoxic signaling intermediates orchestrate a whole host of responses from angiogenesis, glycolysis, and erythropoiesis to inflammation and remodeling, which could be beneficial or harmful to the hosting organ. The length of exposure to low oxygen pressure as well as the existing signaling pathways within different cells dictates their benefit or disadvantage from hypoxic signaling. Therefore, activation or inhibition of hypoxic intermediates could serve as novel therapeutic strategies. In this chapter, we review the role of hypoxic signaling in neurodegenerative, inflammatory, and renal disease states and the emerging therapeutic approaches involving hypoxic signaling.

Keywords: hypoxia, hypoxia-inducible factor, neurodegenerative disease, Parkinson's disease, Alzheimer's disease, ischemia/reperfusion, inflammation, epigenetics, microRNA, inflammatory bowel disease, rheumatoid arthritis, acute kidney injury, chronic kidney disease, erythropoiesis, anemia, allograft rejection

1. Hypoxia and neurodegenerative diseases

1.1. Introduction

Neurodegenerative diseases are defined by the progressive loss of specific neuronal cell population and protein misfolding and aggregate. Reduced oxygen supply has been detected during the aging process as well as the pathogenesis of neurodegenerative diseases. Besides, diseases associated with a lowering of systemic oxygen levels predispose individuals to neurodegenerative diseases. Although the connection between hypoxia and neurodegeneration has been well established, the exact role of hypoxia in neurodegenerative diseases has yet to be elucidated.

This section summarizes current identified clues linking hypoxia to the onset and progression of neurodegenerative diseases, including neurotoxic effects, altered signaling transduction and protein expression, and abnormal epigenetic modification. Furthermore, the following discussion emphasizes on the detrimental impacts of cerebral oxygen deficiency on three major neurodegenerative diseases: Alzheimer's disease (AD), Parkinson's disease (PD), and amyotrophic lateral sclerosis (ALS).

1.1.1. Hypoxia and Alzheimer's disease

AD is characterized by progressive impairments in memory and cognitive function. The hallmark features of AD are extracellular plaques whose major components are amyloid β peptide (Aβ) and intracellular neurofibrillary tangles constituted by hyperphosphorylated tau protein. Other changes identified in AD brains are loss of synapses and neurons, proliferation of reactive astrocytes, and microglial activation. The incidence of AD in the United States is 11% among the population aged over 65 years and approximately 32% among those 85 years and older (Alzheimer's Association, 2015) [1]. Apparently, aging is the most significant risk factor for AD, since the risk of developing AD doubles every 5 years after the age of 65 years. Other factors, including environmental neurotoxins/metals, gene mutations, susceptibility polymorphisms, cardiovascular diseases, traumatic brain injury, and ischemia/hypoxia, also potentially prompt the development of AD.

Although the exact mechanisms and triggers initiating AD remain unclear, both clinical and preclinical studies suggest that hypoxia should be considered as an important risk factor in AD pathogenesis. Chronic cerebral hypoperfusion and glucose hypometabolism appearing decades before cognitive dysfunction promote the initiation and progression of cognitive decline and AD [2]. Patients after cerebral hypoxia or ischemia are more susceptible to developing dementia. Cerebral blood flow (CBF) reduction decreases the synthesis of proteins necessary for memory and learning and contributes likely to neuritic injury, neuronal death, and the onset and progression of dementia [3]. Correspondingly, significantly reduced resting CBF is distinguished in AD patients and is also present in the early stages of AD pathogenesis [4].

Generally, hypoxia modifies Aβ production and tau phosphorylation at numerous points (**Figure 1**). Aβ is a cleavage product generated through the sequential actions of β- and γ-secretases on amyloid precursor protein (APP). Hypoxia can stimulate Aβ generation and senile plaque formation in AD through increasing the expression of β- and γ-secretases along with the localization of γ-secretase from cell body to axon [5]. Furthermore, hypoxia elevates the levels of APP and presenilin-1 (PS-1), a main component of γ-secretase complex, in vivo [6]. The expression of neprilysin (NEP), an enzyme responsible for Aβ degeneration, is reduced during hypoxia [7]. Rats exposed to hypoxic stress display tau hyperphosphorylation in the hippocampus as well as memory deficit, and Aβ-induced tau phosphorylation is raised through calpain upon hypoxia exposure [8, 9]. The activity of protein phosphatase 2A (PP2A) is compromised in AD and is believed to be a cause of tau neurofibrillary. Brain hypoxia generates an acidic environment that promotes the cleavage of I_2^{PP2A}, a potent inhibitor of PP2A, by activating asparaginyl endopeptidase, thus giving rise to tau hyperphosphorylation [10].

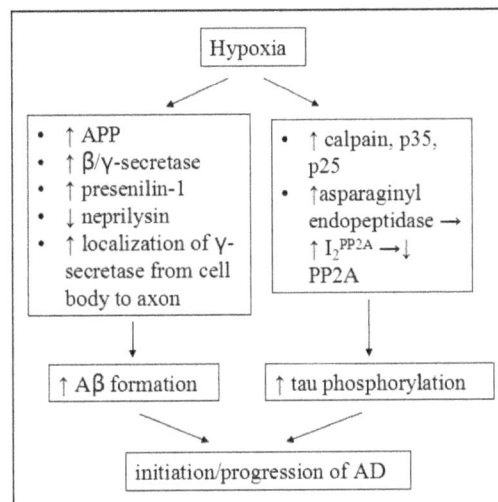

Figure 1. The molecular mechanisms of hypoxic predisposition to AD.

1.1.2. Hypoxia and Parkinson's disease

The clinical features of PD include classical motor symptoms (bradykinesia, rigidity, postural instability, resting tremor) and non-motor symptoms (dementia, sleep disorder, depression, autonomic dysfunction), resulting from a continuous degeneration and loss of dopaminergic neurons in the substantia nigra (SN) and the presence of intracytoplasmic proteinaceous inclusions called Lewy bodies (LB) [11].

α-Synuclein (α-syn), a major constituent of LB, is the pathological hallmark of PD. Hypoxic brain injury is a potential cause of PD, as it enhances α-synuclein expression and aggregation [12]. ATP13A2 (PARK9) mutations have been found in postmortem PD patients, declaring its relevance to PD pathogenesis [13]. Although the exact molecular mechanism remains unknown, it turns out that hypoxia upregulates ATP13A2 transcription via HIF-1 alpha (HIF-1α) in dopaminergic cells [14]. Hypoxia changes the localization of intracellular hemoglobin whose overexpression is correlated with an increased risk of PD [15]. In addition, subnormal sensitivity to hypoxia has been noticed in PD patients even at an early stage of diseases, probably leading to the exacerbation of respiratory failure in PD [16].

1.1.3. Hypoxia and amyotrophic lateral sclerosis

ALS, also known as Lou Gehrig's disease, is a progressive and fetal disease resulted from damaged motor neurons in the spinal cord, brain stem, and motor cortex. The incidence rate of ALS worldwide is estimated to be 2 in 100,000 people, and in the United States, about 5000 persons are diagnosed with ALS every year [17]. ALS risk is influenced by physical activity, smoking habit, type of diet, and exposure to agriculture chemicals and heavy metals. Occupations that may cause intermittent hypoxia, such as fire fighter, double the risk of ALS, and genetic impairment in reaction to hypoxia predisposes motor neuron to death [18].

Hypoxia is not only a causative factor of ALS but also accelerates the progression of ALS. Motor neurons under hypoxic conditions fail to survive and undergo degeneration [19]. SOD1^{G93A} mutant mice, an ALS animal model, have experienced aggravation in motor neuronal loss, neuromuscular weakness and possibly cognitive deficiency, with higher level of oxidative stress and inflammation after chronic intermittent hypoxia [20]. Chronic sustained hypoxic condition induces the activation of apoptosis-related genes such as caspase 3, apoptosis-inducing factor (AIF), and cytochrome C in motor neurons from the spinal cord of ALS mice, facilitating the progression of ALS [21].

1.2. The mechanism of hypoxia-induced injury in neural cells

Cellular and molecular pathways underlying hypoxia-induced neurotoxicity and cell death are multifaceted and complex, including a number of cross-talked mechanisms. Ensuing hypoxia stimulates the production and release of proteins mediating oxidative stress, inflammation, apoptosis, mitochondrial metabolism, metal homeostasis, synaptic transmission, and autophagy, contributing to neuronal death (**Figure 2**).

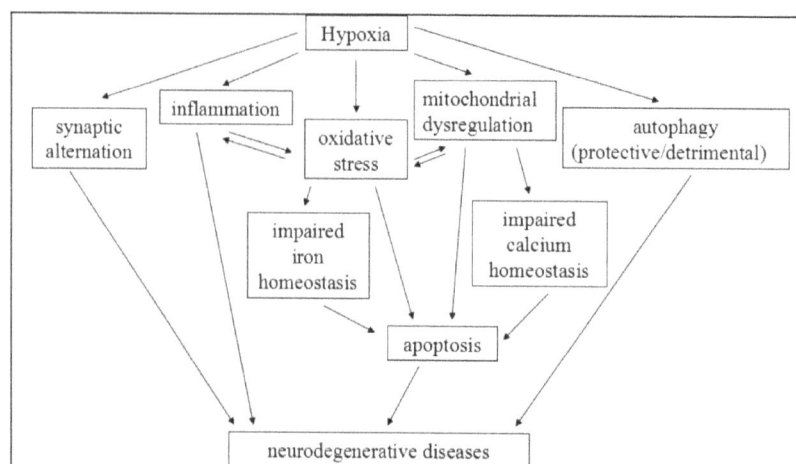

Figure 2. Different pathogenic mechanisms linking hypoxia to neurodegenerative diseases.

1.2.1. Hypoxia-promoted oxidative stress

Oxidative stress has been implicated in hypoxic injury and neurodegenerative diseases. It occurs due to the disruption of oxidative balance and excessive production of reactive oxygen species (ROS) and reactive nitrogen species (RNS), including hydrogen peroxide (H_2O_2), nitric oxide (NO), superoxide (O_2^-), and the highly reactive hydroxyl radicals ($\cdot$OH) [22]. The production of ROS and RNS is increased under hypoxic condition, probably because there is no acceptor for the electrons available. During hypoxic events, high levels of free radicals are produced through mitochondrial complex III, and the antioxidant status is depleted, thus leading to oxidative damage of vital cellular components. For instance, neuroblastoma cells exposed to hypoxia have augmented production of free radicals accompanied by a concomitant decrease in reduced glutathione (GSH) content, glutathione reductase (GR), glutathione peroxidase (GPx), and superoxide dismutase (SOD) activities, further inciting apoptotic death [22].

Increased oxidative stress is believed to be associated with neurological disorders and classical neuropathy. Reduced antioxidant capacity is a trait of AD. The activation of NO/NOS signaling system by cerebral ischemia in aged rats triggers hippocampal Aβ production through β-secretase 1 (BACE1) pathway, implying RNS is a bridge linking hypoxia to AD [23]. In retinal ganglion cells (RGEs) derived from rats, hypoxia exposure triggers Aβ formation, intracellular ROS accumulation, and following cell death, suggesting the involvement of Aβ in hypoxia-induced retinal degeneration in AD [24]. In PD, the promotion of ROS formation is highly correlated to mutant α-syn phosphorylation at serine 129 (Ser129), possibly preceding cell degeneration [25]. Agents with antioxidant property ameliorate neurodegenerative situation, including natural compounds and iron chelators.

1.2.2. Hypoxia-altered ionic homeostasis

Impaired cellular homeostasis of metals can be triggered by hypoxic conditions, resulting in neurodegeneration through various mechanisms, such as oxidative stress, inflammation, and aberrant expression of metalloproteins.

Calcium dyshomeostasis is a fundamental mechanism in the pathogenesis of neurodegenerative diseases. The interaction between γ-aminobutyric acid (GABA) and calcium-dependent neurotransmission as well as calcium-dependent neuronal metabolism also reveals the role of Ca^{2+} in neuronal degeneration. Ca^{2+} acts as an intracellular messenger, controlling not only transsynaptic signal transmission but also cellular metabolism by reaching the mitochondria [26]. Hypoxia can disrupt Ca^{2+} entry and signaling in various cell types. In hypoxic human neuroblastoma cells, the storage of intracellular Ca^{2+}, Na^+/Ca^{2+} exchange, and capacitative Ca^{2+} entry are boosted, indicating adaptive cellular remodeling in response to prolonged hypoxia [27]. Similarly, chronic hypoxia enhances capacitative Ca^{2+} entry and mitochondria Ca^{2+} content in the primary culture of rat type-I cortical astrocytes [28]. In terms of AD, chronic hypoxia potentiates posttranscriptional trafficking of L-type Ca^{2+} channels that may result from the interaction between Aβ and Ca^{2+} channel subunit [29].

Iron can be released from storage protein in the brain under hypoxic circumstances, and disruption of intracellular free iron homeostasis is an early event upon hypoxic stimulation in oligodendrocytes that contain enriched iron and ferritin [30]. Progressive hypoxia dramatically activates the synthesis of ferritin, a major iron-binding protein, in oligodendrocytes, and this induction may require ROS formation as it can be enhanced by co-treatment with H_2O_2 [31]. Intracellular free iron has neurotoxic effects. Iron promotes Aβ aggregation in vitro [32], and iron-Aβ interaction exhibits toxic effects through ROS [33]. Iron also binds to tau, but interestingly, its effect on tau relies on the oxidation state. Fe^{3+} induces the aggregation of hyperphosphorylated tau and reduces the phosphorylation of tau, whereas Fe^{2+} exerts an opposite action [34]. As for PD, abnormal accumulation of iron results in α-syn aggregation by promoting its synthesis and inhibiting its degradation [35].

1.2.3. Hypoxia-disrupted mitochondrial functions

The consequences of mitochondrial dysfunction cover oxidative stress, intracellular Ca^{2+} dysregulation, apoptosis, and metabolic failure, aggravating the deleterious effect.

Respiratory chain reprogramming is the first stage in the development of hypoxia-triggered mitochondrial disorders, converting complex I electron transport chain (ETC) to complex II succinate oxidation. The activation of succinate is regarded as a protective and compensatory mechanism in response to oxygen shortage and preserves the aerobic energy production [36]. Otherwise, the dysregulation of complex I during oxygen deficiency may lead neurons to acute degeneration, characterized by decreased membrane potential, loss of ATP, and respiration disorders caused by abnormal oxidation of nicotinamide adenine dinucleotide (NADH) [37]. The study of mitochondrial genes informs that hypoxia upregulates genes involved in glycolytic pathways, indicating a shift in energy production from oxidative phosphorylation to glycolysis, which converts glucose to pyruvate and eventually lactate. This shift is supported by the observation of elevated brain extracellular lactate concentration in traumatic brain injury (TBI) patients. A cerebral microdialysis study discloses that the neurons in TBI patient are unable to utilize lactate produced by astrocyte through tricarboxylic acid (TCA) cycle, leading to increased lactate/pyruvate ratio [38]. In addition, the ketogenic capacity of cultured astroglia and neurons is augmented under hypoxia, probably because of the susceptibility of pyruvate dehydrogenase to oxygen deprivation [39].

Many rare mitochondrial diseases are actually models of neurodegeneration, such as Leber's hereditary optic neuropathy (LHON) and autosomal dominant optic atrophy (ADOA), and abnormal mitochondrial function has been discovered in several age-related neurodegenerative diseases. Suppression of complex I potentiates tau phosphorylation, pointing out the role of mitochondrial dysfunction in the formation of tangles in AD [40]. During prolonged exposure to hypoxia, ROS production, Aβ accumulation, and Ca^{2+} dyshomeostasis are enhanced through regulation on ETC [41]. The SN of PD patients has reduced activity of mitochondrial complex I, and inhibitors of complex I produce neurological changes similar to PD [42].

1.2.4. Hypoxia-mediated apoptotic cascades

Cerebral hypoxia results in increased activities of caspase-9, caspase-8, and caspase-3 in the cerebral cortex of newborn piglets and enhances cytochrome C expression and caspase-3 activity followed by the induction of apoptosis in neuroblastoma cells. NO induced by hypoxia exerts proapoptotic property through elevating the expression of proteins such as Bax and Bad, leading to APAF-1 activation and consequential activation of caspase-9 and caspase-3, and, on the other hand, through downregulating antiapoptotic proteins of the B-cell lymphoma-2 (Bcl-2) family [22, 43] . Exposure of primary neuron cells from ALS mice to chronic sustained hypoxia results in enhanced cellular apoptosis, suggesting hypoxia could accelerate ALS via neuronal apoptosis [21]. Angiogenin (ANG) is a potent inducer of neovascularization and is responsive to hypoxia. Silence of ANG promotes hypoxic injury-induced motor neuron apoptosis, while exogenous overexpression of ANG has an antiapoptotic function. Mutation of ANG has been identified in ALS patients, proposing the importance of ANG in ALS pathogenesis [44].

Blockage of apoptosis can be neuroprotective. Rasagiline and its derivatives, a group of highly potent irreversible monoamine oxidase (MAO) B inhibitor, exert their anti-Parkinson feature by preventing apoptotic cascades. They activate Bcl-2 and protein kinase C (PKC) and inhibit proapoptosis FAS and Bax against neuronal apoptosis [45]. Treatment of 0.5% isoflurane, an inhaled anesthetic, attenuates caspase-3 activation, BACE upregulation, and Bcl-2 reduction caused by hypoxia in H4 human neuroglioma cells, hinting the neuroprotective effect of isoflurane in AD [46].

1.2.5. Hypoxia-modified synaptic signaling

Synaptic transmission in the central nervous system (CNS) is extremely sensitive to hypoxia, since it requires 30–50% of cerebral oxygen. Decrease in synaptic efficacy occurs very early during hypoxia and is possibly the first response of neurons to ischemic insult.

Oxygen-sensitive ion channels and voltage-gated Ca^{2+} and K^+ channel are activated in response to hypoxia, bringing about changes in excitation and inhibition of neuronal and glial cells [47]. Under hypoxic circumstance, there is an accumulation of adenosine in the extracellular space, due to the increased catabolism of adenosine triphosphate (ATP) into adenosine monophosphate (AMP) [48]. Adenosine is a neurotransmitter inhibiting synaptic transmission, and its effect is mediated by adenosine A1 receptor. The mechanism is that receptor activation stimulates inwardly rectifying K^+ channels, substantially inhibiting Ca^{2+} channels, phospholipase C activation, and the release of neurotransmitters including glutamate, dopamine, serotonin, and acetylcholine [49].

P2Y1 receptor is a G-protein-coupled ATP receptor activated by ATP released from neurons and astrocytes during neuronal activity or under pathophysiological conditions such as hypoxia, brain injury, and AD [50]. Emerging evidence shows that P2Y1 receptor obstructs the release of neurotransmitters and modulates synaptic plasticity in the brain, especially in the prefrontal cortex, hippocampus, and cerebellum, leading to impaired cognitive process [50]. P2Y1 receptors are localized with AD features such as neurofibrillary tangles and neuritic plaques, suggesting the altered distribution of P2Y1 in AD brains [51]. Astrocytic hyperactivity consisting of single-cell transients and Ca^{2+} waves has been observed around Aβ plaques. P2Y1 receptors are strongly expressed by reactive astrocytes, and blockade of P2Y1 receptors can reduce astrocytic hyperactivity back to normal [52].

1.2.6. Hypoxia and autophagy

In general, autophagy is regarded as a survival mechanism, but under severe hypoxia/ischemia, autophagy may cause self-digestion and eventual cell death due to its overactivation [53]. The morphological characteristics of autophagic-programmed cell death have been observed in both mice and rats with cerebral ischemia [54, 55].

Enormous studies indicate autophagy dysfunction in AD. Autophagic vacuoles (AVs) are significantly accumulated in the brain of AD patients compared to normal brain, possibly leading to lysosomal enzyme dysfunction [56]. The cross talk between autophagy and tau aggregation indicates the change of autophagic function in the pathogenesis of AD. Autophagy initially degrades tau to protect neurons; however, hyperphosphorylation of tau results in autophagic dysfunction, which substantially exacerbates AD via inducing tau aggregation [57, 58]. Remarkably, hypoxia induces autophagic activation through AMPK-mTOR signaling, resulting in more Aβ production and AD aggravation in vitro [56].

Defective autophagy has been implicated in PD [59], and several mutations in PD are strongly relevant to autophagy dysregulation, such as PTEN-induced putative kinase 1 (PINK1) [60]. Autophagy in ALS prevents neurons from degeneration, and inhibition of autophagy aggravates motor neuron viability, since the aggregates composed of intermediate filaments and insoluble forms of proteins can be cleared by autophagy pathway [61].

1.3. The role of hypoxia-sensitive transcription factors in neurodegenerative diseases

Several transcription factors are responsive to hypoxia and subsequently alter gene expression and cellular activity. The signaling pathways relevant to these transcription factors have been indicated in the development of neurodegenerative diseases. Therefore, these transcription factors may provide a link between hypoxic environment and neurodegeneration. The following discussion will include HIF-1, the most well-studied hypoxia-inducible gene, and two other redox-sensitive transcription factors, nuclear factor-kappa B (NF-κB) and NF-E2-related factor 2 (Nrf2).

1.3.1. Hypoxia-inducible factor-1

Hypoxia-inducible factor-1 (HIF-1) is a transcriptional activator involved in oxygen hemostasis, regulating the expression of genes and the activation of signaling pathways that participate in angiogenesis, erythropoiesis, neovascularization, iron metabolism, glucose metabolism, cell proliferation, apoptosis, and cell cycle control (**Figure 3**).

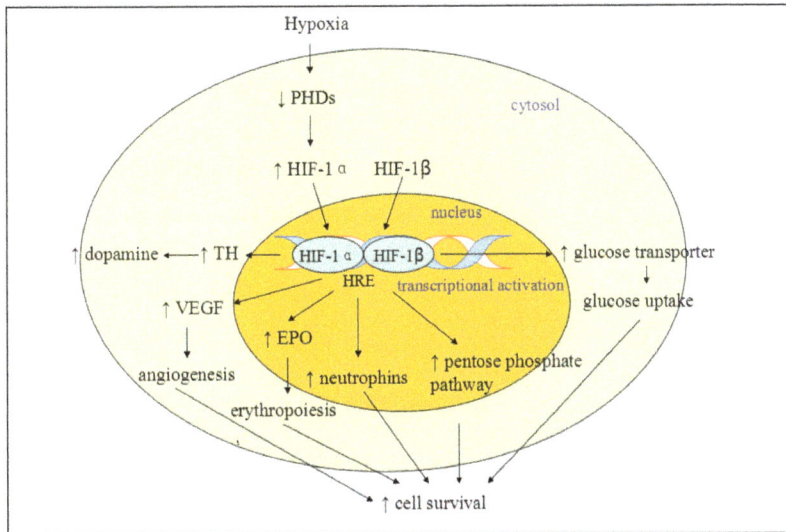

Figure 3. The neuroprotective role of HIF-1α activation in hypoxia.

In AD, HIF-1α upregulates neuronal glucose transporters such as GLUT-1 and GLUT-3 and facilitates glucose uptake, thus providing increased oxygen supply to hypoxic tissues [62]. It also contributes to cell survival by inducing the key enzymes in pentose phosphate pathway, including glucose-6-phosphate dehydrogenase and 6-phosphogluconate dehydrogenase [63]. HIF-1α also connects hypoxia to amyloidogenic processing of APP through transcriptionally upregulating BACE1 and eventually increases Aβ formation [64].

The protective role of HIF-1 in PD has been demonstrated by its ability to increase dopamine synthesis and dopaminergic neuron growth. Tyrosine hydroxylase (TH) is the rate-limiting enzyme of dopamine synthesis in dopaminergic neurons, and interestingly, it contains an HRE [65]. HIF-1 elevated in response to hypoxia increases TH expression in rat brain stem, and HIF-1α conditional knockout mice exhibit reduced expression of TH and aldehyde dehydrogenase in SN [57]. HIF-1 activation may defend against dysregulation of brain iron homeostasis and mitochondria in PD. Iron accumulation has been observed in the SN of PD patients and is considered as a culprit of ROS generation and intracellular α-syn aggregation [66]. Moreover, the neurotransmitter dopamine is a metal reductant that reduces the oxidation state of metals such as Fe^{3+} and subsequently results in elevated oxidative stress [67]. Deferoxamine (DFO), an iron chelator, prevents neurotoxicity in MPTP-treated mice through upregulation of HIF-1α protein expression, leading to declined expression of proteins such as α-syn, divalent metal transporter with iron-responsive element (DMT1 + IRE) and transferrin receptor (TFR), and elevated expression of HIF-1 target genes, including TH, vascular endothelial growth factor (VEGF), and growth associated protein 43 (GAP43) [68].

HIF-1 activation during hypoxia should be beneficial to ALS. HIF-1-VEGF pathway can induce angiogenesis and increase blood supply to motor neurons. VEGF overexpression delays motor neuron loss and impairment in SOD1^{G93A} mutant mice and prolongs the survival of mice [69]. Deletion of HRE in VEGF promoter region abolishes hypoxia-increased VEGF expression, causing motor neuron degeneration [70]. Additionally, HIF-1-erythropoietin (EPO) pathway is suggested to be a new therapeutic target for ALS. EPO treatment in SOD1^{G93A} mice postpones the onset and progression of motor deterioration and modulates the immune-inflammatory response through reducing the levels of pro-inflammatory cytokines and enhancing the expression of anti-inflammatory cytokines [71, 72]. However, both above pathways are impaired in ALS. The level of VEGF is low in the CSF of early ALS patients, and likewise, the expression of VEGF in the CSF from hypoxemic ALS patients is lower than that in the CSF from normoxemic ALS patients [73, 74]. EPO protein level is declined in the surrounding glial cells of SOD1^{G93A} mice, and in the anterior horn cells (AHCs) from SOD1^{G93A} mice, impaired cytoplasmic-nuclear transport of HIF-1α has appeared since the presymptomatic stage, indicating the abnormality in HIF-1 pathway might precede motor neuron degradation [75, 76].

The well-studied group of agents targeting HIF-1 is iron chelators. The neuroprotective and neurorestorative activities of M30, an iron chelator with brain-selective monoamine oxidase (MAO) AB inhibitory function, share a same pathway, the activation of HIF-1, in different neurodegenerative diseases. M30 elevates HIF-1 to regulate neurotrophins BDNF, GDNF, VEGF, and EPO in PD, and meanwhile, it delays the onset of ALS in SOD1^{G93A} mutant mice through HIF-1 upregulation [77, 78]. In APP/PS1 AD mice model, M30 treatment upregulates HIF-1α in the frontal cortex, resulting in the beneficial modulation of target glycolytic gene expression, such as aldolase A, enolase-1, and GLUT-1 [79].

Taken together, HIF-1 is a key player protecting neuron cells against hypoxia and oxidative stress, as well as a reasonable therapeutic target against major neurodegenerative diseases, since its participation in the pathogenesis of neurodegeneration has been well identified.

1.3.2. Nuclear factor-kappa B

Nuclear factor-kappa B (NF-κB) is analogous to HIF-1 in structure, function, and mechanism of activation and plays a critical role in inflammation, immune response, synaptic transmission, neuronal plasticity, and apoptosis [80]. In resting state, NF-κB is complexed with the inhibitory subunit I-κB; however, under physiological or pharmacological stimulus such as oxidative stress, I-kappa B (I-κB) is degraded, leading to translocation of NF-κB from cytoplasm to nucleus to modulate gene transcription. NF-κB and I-κB proteins comprise a growing family of structurally related transcription factors, and functional NF-κB complexes are present in generally all cell types in the nervous system, such as neurons, astrocytes, microglia, and oligodendrocytes [81, 82]. In neurons, the most common variants consist of p50, p65/RelA, and I-κB subunits.

As a redox-sensitive transcription factor, the mobilization and upregulation of NF-κB have been reported in hypoxia and ischemia-reperfusion damage. Hypoxic-ischemic brain damage (HIBD) upregulates the expression of NF-κB and the NO content in rat cortex cells, suggesting the involvement of NF-κB/nNOS pathway during the recovery of HIBD-induced neuron damage [83]. The role of NF-κB in neonatal HIBD depends on the duration of hypoxia. Early activation of NF-κB is detrimental, and at that time point, treatment of NF-κB inhibitor, TAT-NBD, exhibits significant therapeutic outcomes, whereas late NF-κB activation enhances antiapoptotic pathway and contributes to endogenous neuroprotection [84]. The overall effect of NF-κB activation seems to facilitate ischemic neuronal degeneration, but still, the effect can be either neuroprotective or deleterious depending on the cell type and the strength of signal [85]. The suppression of NF-κB or I-κB in neuron can reduce infarct size after stroke, and the inhibition of NF-κB caused by Ginkgolide B has protective effects on ischemic stroke [86, 87].

NF-κB activation has been observed in neurons and astroglia of brain sections from AD patients but only in cells surrounding early plaques, suggesting that the induction of NF-κB activity by Aβ is partially responsible for the aberrant gene expression in diseased nervous tissue [88]. In addition, intraperitoneal injection of sodium hydrosulfide (NaHS), a donor of H_2S whose level is reduced in the hippocampus of Aβ-injected rats, inhibits MAPK/NF-κB pathway and dramatically mitigates cognitive decline and neuroinflammation [83]. Another novel drug for AD, Gx-50, exerts anti-inflammatory effects against Aβ-triggered microglial overactivation in AD mice model via inhibition of NF-κB signaling [89].

Increased NF-κB activation has been reported in dopaminergic neurons of SN from PD patients, as well as in astrocytes of spinal cords from ALS patients [90]. Compounds inhibiting NF-κB translocation in microglia such as vinyl sulfone compound (VSC2) downregulate the expression of inducible NOS (iNOS) and TNF-α, leading to anti-inflammatory and antioxidant events in PD animal model [91]. NF-κB is also involved in microglia-induced motor neuron death in ALS. Deletion of NF-κB signaling in microglia rescues motor neuron from microglia-mediated death and extends survival in ALS mice by impairing pro-inflammatory microglial activation [92].

Collectively, NF-κB is responsive to the injury of nervous system in both acute and chronic neurodegenerative conditions. Agents suppressing NF-κB activation have been tested in animal models of neurodegenerative conditions, but their usage should be considered cautiously because of the involvement of NF-κB in learning and memory.

1.3.3. NF-E2-related factor 2

NF-E2-related factor 2 (Nrf2) is a basic leucine zipper (bZIP) transcription factor that is ubiquitously expressed in a wide range of tissues and cell types. It heterodimerizes with small Maf or Jun proteins and binds to the antioxidant response element (ARE) in the promoter region of target genes in response to oxidative stress [93]. Nrf2 knockout mice are susceptible to oxidative stress and neurodegeneration without obvious phenotypic defects [94].

The upregulation of Nrf2 exerts neuroprotective action during hypoxia/ischemia. Hypoxia preconditioning on rat brain against severe hypoxia or ischemia insult is through upregulating Nrf2 and HO-1 expression and alleviating oxidative stress damage [95]. rhEPO administration in ischemic rat activates Keap-Nrf2/ARE pathway to decrease H_2O_2 concentration and to protect brain tissue [96]. Similarly, in oxygen-deficient astrocytes, sulfiredoxin-1, an endogenous antioxidant protein, ameliorates oxidative stress via Nrf2/ARE pathway to prevent the brain from ischemic injury [97].

The expression level of Nrf2 is significantly decreased in the hippocampal neurons from AD patients [98]. The beneficial effect of Nrf2 upregulation in AD is evidenced by the finding that Nrf2 is able to induce NDP52, an autophagy adaptor protein, which facilitates the clearance of phosphorylated tau in neurons [99]. Examination of postmortem brain samples from PD patients reveals that NQO1 and p62 whose expression is associated with Nrf2 are partly sequestered in LB, demonstrating the impaired Nrf2 signaling in PD, and pharmacological activation of Nrf2 defends PD by protecting nigral dopaminergic neurons against α-syn toxicity and decreasing astrocytosis and microgliosis [100]. Correspondingly, in ALS mice model, WN1316, a novel acylaminoimidazole, boosts the activity of Nrf2 to protect motor neurons against oxidative injury and repress glial inflammation, microgliosis, and astrocytosis [101].

The Nrf2 signaling pathway is an attractive therapeutic target for neurodegenerative diseases, and thus, the chemopreventive agents aiming at Nrf2 might be suitable candidates against the development and progression of neurodegeneration.

1.4. Epigenetic modification

Epigenetics is the study of heritable and nonheritable changes in gene expression without changes to the underlying DNA sequence. Currently, at least three systems, DNA methylation, histone medication, and noncoding RNA (ncRNA)-associated gene silencing, are identified in epigenetic changes. A large body of evidence documents that hypoxia triggers epigenetic alternation that contributes to the initiation and aggravation of neurodegeneration.

1.4.1. Modification of DNA and histone

DNA methylation and histone modification are two important epigenetic mechanisms altering the transcription of genes. The methylation of CpG island in the promoter region results in the silence of gene expression, whereas demethylation undergoes the opposite direction. The posttranslational modification (PTM) of histone includes acetylation, methylation, and phosphorylation that are regulated by pairs of enzymes, impacting gene expression via altering chromatin structure or recruiting histone modifiers.

Short-term hypoxia causes long-lasting changes in genomic DNA methylation in hippocampal neuronal cells and subsequent alternation in the expression of a number of genes participating in neural growth and development [102]. Chronic hypoxia-mediated downregulation of NEP in mouse primary cortical and hippocampal neurons is through G9a histone methyltransferase and histone deacetylase 1 (HDAC1) other than methylation of gene promoter [103]. Cultured astrocytes under ischemia-hypoxia (IH) condition show hypermethylation of global DNA and hypoacetylation of histone H3/H4, manifesting epigenetic reprogramming induced by hypoxia [104]. Chronic hypoxia exaggerated the neuropathology and cognitive impairment in AD mice through decreasing the expression of DNA methyltransferase 3b (DNMT3b) to prevent the methylation of γ-secretase promoter [105].

Epigenetic modifications are reversible that make it a promising candidate for therapy. Valproic acid is a neuroprotective agent showing HDAC inhibitory property. It prevents the decrease of H3-Ace in the NEP promoter regions in prenatal hypoxia-induced AD neuropathology, upregulating NEP to improve learning deficits and decrease Aβ level [106].

1.5. Conclusion

This section reviews the major consequences of hypoxia in the CNS and the contribution of individual consequence to the pathogenesis of several neurodegenerative diseases. However, the cross-link among these consequences and how they may predispose hypoxic patients to neurodegeneration remain to be determined, as well as the communication between neurons and glia in response to hypoxic environment. Different types of hypoxia, acute, chronic, sustained, or intermittent, may vary in terms of their effects on neural cells. Therefore, further investigation is required. The prevention of hypoxic condition is clearly helpful for the reduction of neurodegeneration, and the molecules targeted by hypoxia provide therapeutic strategies and interventions against common neurodegenerative diseases.

2. Hypoxia and the inflammatory diseases

2.1. Introduction

Inflammatory diseases are pathological conditions associated with local or systemic activation and persistent activity of inflammatory mediators, leading to cellular, tissue, or organ damage. The inflammatory cascade leads to increased vascular leakage, recruitment of leukocytes, increased generation and secretion of local and systemic inflammatory cytokines and chemokines, and activation and proliferation of innate and adaptive immune cell members. Ultimately, the inflammatory response leads to destruction of target molecules as well as their hosting cells and tissues, which could lead to pathological conditions such as inflammatory bowel disease and rheumatoid arthritis.

Hypoxia and inflammation have been extensively studied, and the two conditions seem to have a complex interrelated relationship. In general, hypoxia induces the inflammatory response via activation of cytokines and inflammatory cells, while inflammatory states are complemented with severe hypoxia and induction of hypoxic signaling intermediates [107, 108]. A key mediator of hypoxic signaling in inflammation is HIF-1. Aside from low oxygen tension, recent evidence shows that various oxygen-independent pathways regulate HIF-1α transcription and translation under normoxia. For example, endogenous nitric oxide has been shown to stabilize HIF-1α under normoxia [109–111]. Angiotensin II is another factor that increases HIF-1α transcription and translation under normoxia, and angiotensin receptor blockade has shown to independently reduce HIF-1α levels under hypoxic injury [112, 113]. Other nonhypoxic HIF-1 regulatory molecules are via growth factors, thrombin, bacterial lipopolysaccharide (LPS), interleukins, and tumor necrosis factor-α (TNF-α) [114]. In general transcriptional and translational regulation of HIF-1α occurring as a secondary mode of HIF-1 regulation may aggravate or hinder the hypoxic response of the protein.

It has been noted that during hypoxemic states the levels of inflammatory cytokines such as IL-1, IL6, and TNF-α increase in serum [107, 115, 116]. Activation of macrophages and other innate and adaptive immune cell members is also shown to be induced by HIF-1 under hypoxia via activation of Toll-like receptor (TLR) signaling [117, 118]. Likewise, ischemia reperfusion is associated with recruitment of polymorphonuclear (PMN) leukocytes and vascular leakage [116, 119, 120]. This response is shown to be mediated via several endothelial cell surface glycoproteins and receptors and secondary activation of signaling via HIF-1–induced adenosine generation and NF-κB [116, 119].

It is noteworthy that ischemia and hypoxia are observed in inflamed tissues due to occlusion of blood flow via inflammatory cells [108]. As a result, signaling via inflammatory intermediates has been shown to potentiate hypoxic signaling via HIF-1. Macrophages in specific have been shown to release cytokines that stabilize and increase the activity of HIF-1 [111, 121]. Ultimately, transcriptional activation of factors such as VEGF by HIF-1 seems to increase angiogenesis and blood flow restoration to the site of inflammation.

Activation of HIF-1 further assures energy supply and survival of myeloid cells as well as bactericidal capacity of macrophages [122, 123]. Among the signaling pathways induced by HIF-1 in macrophages are mediators such as NF-κB, TNF-α, and nitric oxide that play key roles in the inflammatory capacity of the myeloid cells [111, 121, 123]. Interestingly, HIF-1α stabilization in turn positively regulates the production of inflammatory cytokines such as TNF-α, and therefore, through a positive feedback mechanism, inflammation and hypoxic signaling potentiate one another [123]. In the following sections, detailed mechanisms of this interaction will be discussed. Furthermore, the role of hypoxia and HIF molecules in arthritic and inflammatory bowel disease (IBD) pathophysiology and potential therapeutic targets relating to hypoxic signaling will be examined.

2.2. Hypoxic signaling and key inflammatory intermediates

2.2.1. TNF-α

TNF-α is a key mediator of the inflammatory response. It has been shown that HIF-1a stabilization and DNA-binding activity are enhanced by TNF-α [111]. Interaction of TNF-α and HIF-1 is rather complex. Physiologically, the stabilization of HIF-1a by TNF-α is thought to be mediated by activated macrophages [121]. Accumulation of HIF-1α via the TNF-α is via a mechanism independent from hypoxic accumulation or transcriptional activation of HIF-1α. Several studies have investigated the mechanism of HIF-1α stabilization via TNF-α, and among such mechanisms, NF-κB signaling seems to be the key mediator of this process [124, 125]. Studies by Zhou et al. have shown that TNF-α leads to accumulation of ubiquitinated form of HIF-1α, which is normally one of HIF-1α degradation steps. This interaction was mediated through increased NF-κB transcription [124]. They also noted that transfection of cells with p50/p65 members of NF-κB family leads to normoxic accumulation of HIF-1α in the absence of TNF-α [124]. Interestingly it has also been shown that reactive oxygen species (ROS) such as H_2O_2 or SO^- interfere with TNF-α–mediated accumulation of HIF-1α [126]. Aside from protein accumulation, additional studies have shown increased translation of HIF-1α via TNF-α that is also mediated via NF-κB through upregulation of an antiapoptotic protein Bcl-2 [127].

2.2.2. Nuclear factor-kappa β

NF-κB is a family of transcription factors involved in development, proliferation, survival, and antimicrobial response of innate and adaptive immune system cells. Numerous extensive studies have been conducted to elucidate the very complex role of NF-κB in the immune response [128]. The NF-κB family is composed of five related transcription factors, which can form homodimers or heterodimer complexes with DNA-binding activity. These identified members are p50, p52, RelA (p65), RelB, and c-Rel [128]. NF-κB complexes are inactive in the cytoplasm and are bound to an inhibitory protein called I-κB. Once NF-κB signaling is activated, the I-κB proteins are degraded, which then allow the transcription factors to translocate to the nucleus [128]. In the innate immune response, NF-κB is activated secondary to Toll-like receptor (TLR) activation. Toll-like receptors are pattern recognition receptors (PRR), which help immune cells recognize and combat pathogenic components. There are 11 identified mammalian TLRs with various coupled signaling pathways. TLRs are expressed in the cytosol as well as on the plasma membrane of immune cells [128]. Upon ligand binding, TLR signaling leads to recruitment of specific adaptor proteins and second messenger molecules, which in turn activate several transcription factors. Among such signaling pathways are mediators that result in degradation of I-κB proteins and activation of NF-κB [128]. NF-κB in turn induces gene expression of cytokines and other proteins involved in bactericidal activity against pathogens. NF-κB activation and signaling are also involved in adaptive immunity. T-cell and B-cell receptor activation and signaling activate NF-κB, which in turn activates antiapoptotic proteins and increases transcription of cytokines that ensure survival, proliferation, and differentiation of B and T cells [128].

2.2.3. Hypoxia and the cross talk between HIF-1 and NF-κB

It has been shown that NF-κB is directly activated under hypoxic conditions [129, 130]. Although the mechanism of NF-κB activation under hypoxia remains to be an extensive area of research, it has been shown that I-κB tyrosine residues are phosphorylated under hypoxia [129]. More recent studies suggest phosphorylation and inactivation of I-κB under hypoxia occur secondary to activation of transforming growth factor beta-activated kinase-1 (TAK1) and I-kappa B kinase (IKK) complex, primarily responsible for in I-κB degradation resulting in NF-κB activation [130–133]. Additionally, it has been shown that O_2-dependent prolyl hydroxylases (PHDs) that are involved in HIF-1 inactivation also play a role in proline hydroxylation of IKKβ and NF-κB repression [133]. Thus, during hypoxia loss of PHD activity would activate NF-κB.

Although hypoxic activation of NF-κB is to be better understood, a large body of convincing evidence shows a critical role for NF-κB in induction of HIF-1. Activation of NF-κB leads to induction of HIF-1α gene expression and basal HIF-1α mRNA, and protein levels are dependent upon NF-κB subunit expression levels [134, 135]. Several studies have explored the mechanism of regulation of HIF-1 by NF-κB [124, 127, 134, 136, 137]. It has been shown that NF-κB induces expression and increases protein levels of HIF-1α both in hypoxia and normoxia [124, 134, 137]. Indeed, certain studies suggest that HIF-1α gene expression under hypoxia is dependent upon intact NF-κB signaling pathway [134, 137]. These studies also provide mechanistic evidence into the regulation of HIF-1α gene expression via binding of several NF-κB subunits to the HIF-1α promoter region [134, 135]. Thus, secondary to direct activation of HIF-1 under hypoxic conditions, interaction of NF-κB additionally contributes to this process by increasing basal levels of HIF-1α protein.

Respective regulation of NF-κB by HIF-1 has also been reported in the literature [114, 138, 139]. These studies suggest direct activation of NF-κB via HIF-1 signaling in inflammatory cells. Among suggested mechanisms are increased expression of TLR2 and TLR6 leading to activation of NF-κB, hyperphosphorylation of IKKβ, and phosphorylation of serine residues of p65 subunit of NF-κB leading to its translocation to nucleus and transcriptional activity [117, 138, 139].

Overall, hypoxia and signaling via NF-κB and HIF-1 are closely linked and, respectively, regulate one another to enhance the inflammatory response.

2.3. Hypoxia and inflammatory bowel disease (IBD)

IBD is associated with loss of intestinal mucosal barrier, inflammation of mucosa, and increased incidence of bacterial infections [140]. IBD is categorized as ulcerative colitis (UC) and Crohn's disease (CD). Both conditions are associated with severe inflammation and breakdown of intestinal mucosal barrier and chronic gastrointestinal discomfort. Current therapeutic approaches to IBD include anti-inflammatory agents mostly targeted at TNF-α and immune cell members.

Hypoxia has been shown to be a critical component of inflammation in IBD. Surgical specimens of intestinal mucosa of IBD patients show increased expression of HIF-1 and HIF-2 [141]. Increased vascular proliferation and density has been noted in intestines of IBD patients secondary to hypoxia-induced VEGF activity [142]. Additionally microvascular abnormality and loss of endothelial nitric oxide production are seen in IBD mucosa [143].

The intestinal mucosa is exposed to fluctuating levels of oxygen. On the one hand, the intestinal lumen is nearly anoxic, and oxygen pressure is generally low on the luminal side of the mucosa. On the other hand, the rate of perfusion of the subendothelium is dependent upon meal intake, and PO_2 changes dramatically from high to low in between meals. The shift in oxygen tension in the mucosal layer renders it resistant to hypoxic states. This could be in part due to basal activity of hypoxic signaling intermediates such as HIF-1 in the intestinal mucosal. Indeed, HIF-1α–null mice in the intestinal epithelium show diminished mucosal protection and increased clinical symptoms in murine model of colitis [144]. HIF-1–induced epithelial protection is shown to be due to induction of several proteins such as mucin, p-glycoprotein, and ecto-5′-nucleotidase (CD73), an enzyme that converts AMP to adenosine (A_2B) receptor [140]. Adenosine production during hypoxia has shown to decrease vascular leakage and neutrophil accumulation and thus plays an anti-inflammatory role [120]. In a case-control cohort study, patients with polymorphisms in CD39, a vascular and immune cell ecto-nucleotidase that converts extracellular ATP and ADP to AMP, had increased susceptibility to Crohn's disease [145]. Therefore, HIF-1 signaling via adenosine is a key step in protection against IBD inflammation (**Figure 4**).

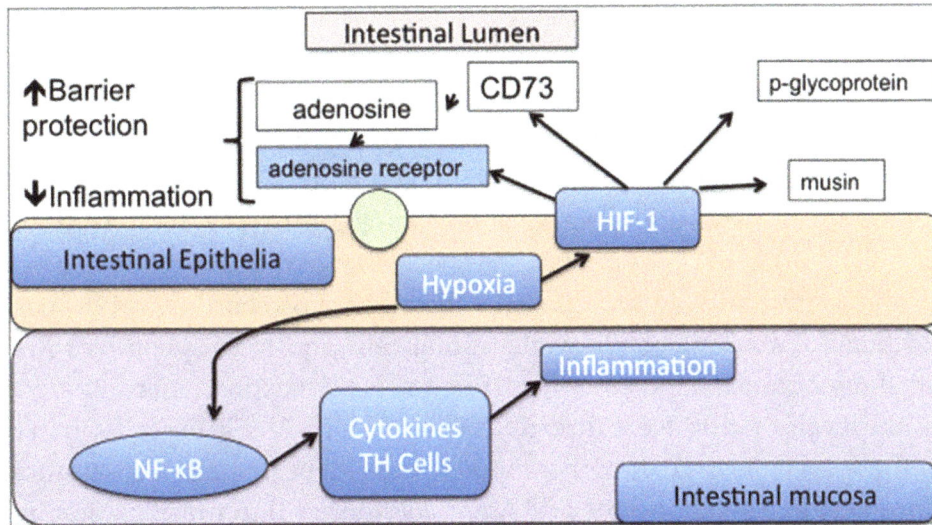

Figure 4. Hypoxia and IBD pathogenesis.

Aside from HIF-1, NF-κB is also involved in inflammatory events of IBD [146, 147]. Nuclear levels of NF-κB p65 have long been seen in lamina propria biopsies of patients with Crohn's disease [148]. Activation of NF-κB in mucosal macrophages leads to induction of pro-inflammatory cytokines such as TNF-α, IL-1, and IL-6, which mediate mucosal tissue damage [149]. NF-κB activation in intestinal mucosa also plays a role in differentiation of T-helper cells, which also play a role in IBD inflammation (**Figure 4**) [149]. In addition to pro-inflammatory activity, some studies have shown a protective role for NF-κB [146]. Loss of β or γ subunits of the IKK complex leads to colitis and apoptosis of intestinal mucosa [150, 151]. Additionally, polymorphisms of TLR4 and TLR5, which are involved in NF-κB activation, have been strongly associated with IBD in canines [152]. The protective role of NF-κB in IBD is thought to be in terms of maintaining mucosal barrier and integrity. Overall, NF-κB seems to play a dual role in IBD.

Due to the protective role of HIF-1 in models of colitis, it has been proposed that induction of HIF-1 could serve as a potential therapeutic target for treatment of IBD. The common pharmacological method of HIF-1 induction is via inhibition of PHD enzymes, which break down the HIF-1α subunit in the presence of oxygen. In vitro pharmacological inhibition of PHD using 2-oxoglutarate analogs as co-substrates of PHDs or dimethyloxaloglycine, has shown to stabilize HIF-1α [153–155]. In these studies PHD inhibitors decreased clinical symptoms in murine models of colitis and thus present promising therapeutic targets for IBD [153, 155, 156]. As mentioned previously blockade of PHDs can also lead to NF-κB activation. Using PHD inhibitors has thus been suggested to have dual benefits in treatment of IBD.

NF-κB activity, however, is associated with increased inflammation, and therefore, inhibition of NF-κB has also been examined and shows promise in treatment of IBD [149]. Selective NF-κB inhibitors, antisense oligonucleotides against NF-κB, and targeting DNA-binding activity of NF-κB using decoy oligodeoxynucleotides have been among the strategies tested that have produced promising results in murine models of colitis and IBD [157, 158].

2.4. Hypoxia and rheumatoid arthritis (RA)

Rheumatoid arthritis is the most common type of inflammatory arthritis. As an autoimmune disorder, RA is characterized as inflammation of the synovium, loss of cartilage, and bone erosion leading to joint pain and dysfunction [159]. The synovial fluid in RA is infiltrated with fibroblasts, immune cells, and angiogenesis of new vasculature [159, 160]. Additionally, a key feature of synovial fluid in RA is hypoxia. It has been shown that the synovium of knee joints of RA patients has significantly less O_2 pressure than that of osteoarthritis (OA) patients [161]. Immunohistochemical analysis of synovial stromal cells and macrophages of RA- and OA-affected joints show significant increases in HIF1α and HIF2α expression compared to normal. Additionally, the levels of HIFs were directly correlated with VEGF expression in the stromal cell lining in these specimens [162]. Other studies have identified HIF-2α significantly upregulated in fibroblast-like synoviocytes of RA and associated IL-6 upregulation in these cells [163]. These and other similar studies imply HIF signaling as the orchestrator of synovial inflammation and secondary joint damage [159, 164, 165]. A large number of HIF-activated inflamamtory mediators have been identified in RA synovial fluid including but not limited to stromal cell–derived factor 1 (SDF-1), VEGF, TNF-α, IL-1β, and IL-8 [166]. Various TLRs are also expressed in synovial tissue and macrophages, which further activate NF-κB pathway and increase expression of other inflammatory proteins [167]. Not surprisingly, HIF-dependent pathways have also been implicated in TLR expressions in many tissues including synovial cells [117, 118]. Finally, recruitment of CXCR4+ lymphocytes and matrix metalloproteinases (MMPs) in the synovial fibroblasts involved in cartilage destruction has also shown to be HIF-1 mediated and NF-κB mediated [168, 169]. Overall, a large body of evidence implicates hypoxia and HIF signaling as a key underlying mechanism in pathogenesis of RA (**Figure 5**).

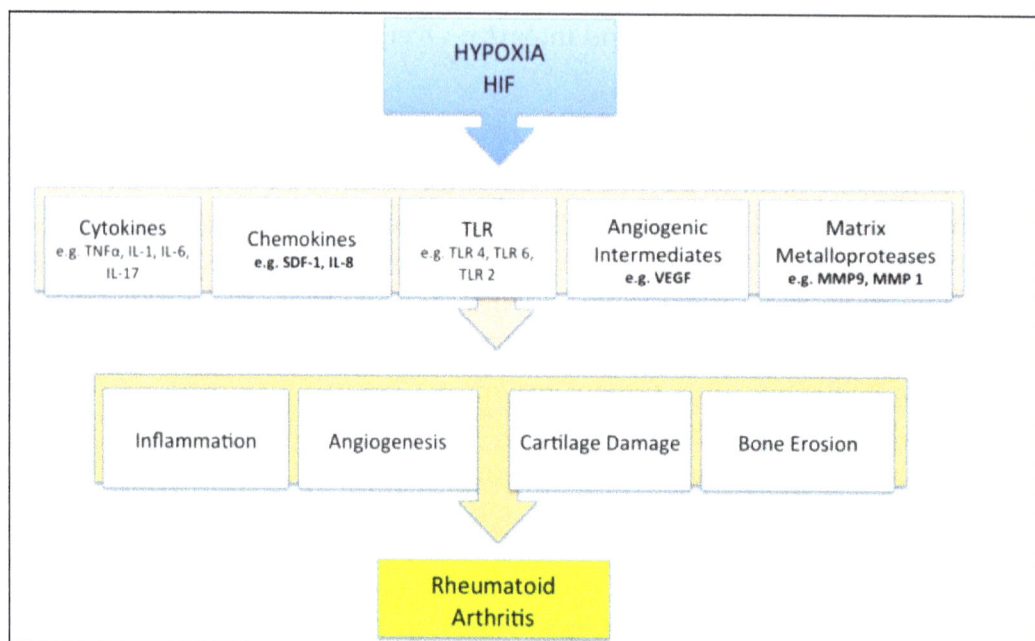

Figure 5. Hypoxia and pathogenesis of rheumatoid arthritis.

As discussed above, hypoxia- and HIF-mediated signaling is highly pro-inflammatory and destructive in RA. The key approach to treatment of RA is thus inhibition of HIF signaling. Many HIF inhibitors have been tested in cancer that may show promise in treatment of RA [170]. The limiting factor in administering HIF inhibitors is pharmacokinetic availability of these compounds in the synovial space as well as specific targetting of joints rather than systemic therapy. Gene targetting of HIF molecules using antisense oligonucleotides targetting HIF-1α mRNA has also been tested, which may show efficacy in RA treatment [159]. Additional approaches including anti-VEGF antibodies or anti-VEGF receptor molecules have been tested in models of arthritis and have shown efficacy in delaying onset and severity of RA in animal models [159, 171]. These strategies remain to be clinically tested yet show great promise in novel therapeutics of RA.

2.5. Conclusion

Section 2 discussed the complex relationship between hypoxia and inflammatory process and highlighted the key intermediates and pathways involved in this relationship. The discovery of hypoxic-inflammatory pathways has led to a greater understanding of inflammatory and autoimmune diseases such as IBD and RA and the use of novel pharmacological approaches targetting HIF and hypoxic signaling intermediates in these conditions. So far, these agents have been mostly studied in cancer clinical trials. Additional clinical studies are needed to examine the safety and efficacy of new HIF-modulating agents in treatment of inflammatory disease states.

3. Hypoxia and renal diseases

3.1. Introduction

Approximately 26 million Americans have some evidence of chronic kidney disease (CKD) and are at risk to develop kidney failure. The number of Americans with end-stage renal diseases (ESRD) is expected to grow to 785,000 by 2020 (currently 485,000). The annual cost of treating ESRD is currently over $32 billion. It is estimated that healthcare system can save up to $18.5 to $60.6 billion by reducing rate of progression of chronic kidney disease (CKD) by 10–30% over the next decade.

In acute setting acute kidney injury (AKI) has been shown to be associated with bad outcome, for instance, mortality rate of hospitalized patients with AKI increases more than fourfold [172]. Due to high medical and economic impact of AKI and CKD, finding new therapeutic tools in treatment of CKD is becoming of an increasing importance.

Hypoxia-inducible factor (HIF) has become the focus of medical community as a putative target because its augmentation is likely to ease the burden of kidney disease. The following sections discuss the evidence regarding the role of HIF molecules in various kidney pathologies and potential therapeutic approaches with respect to the HIF system.

3.1.1. Pathophysiology

Kidneys have a rich blood supply. In fact human kidneys receive 20% of cardiac output, while they weigh less than 1% of the total body weight. However, renal medulla, physiologically, has low oxygen tension and hence is very sensitive to hypoxia.

Hypoxia is the final common pathway to irreversible renal damage and eventually ESRD [173]. Since Fine et al. introduced chronic hypoxia hypothesis for the first time, it has been confirmed in several studies [174]. Also, hypoxia plays a role in pathogenesis of AKI as well as transformation of AKI to CKD.

Three phases of cell damage have been recognized following hypoxic insult to kidneys (by ligation of a branch of renal artery) [175]:

• Phase I: 1–6 h post hypoxic damage; in this phase parenchymal cells still appear viable.

• Phase II or intermediate phase: 1–3 days following insult; in this phase tissue damage is completed.

• Phase III or late phase: after 3 days; when tissue repair and remodeling are initiated.

In order to survive hypoxemia or regional hypoxia, the kidneys adopt a set of sophisticated defense mechanisms, which include expression of HIF. HIF is the cornerstone of adaptation to hypoxia. This master regulator of the cellular response to hypoxia orchestrates several hundred target genes affecting metabolism, the cell cycle, and inflammation [176]. The hypoxia-inducible transcription factors have been extensively studied in the kidneys [177]. HIF-1α is mainly expressed in tubular cells, while HIF-2α is found in peritubular, interstitial, endothelial, and glomerular regions [178]. Likewise, PHD1 and PHD3 are mostly present in glomeruli, and PHD1, PHD2, and PHD3 express more in the distal tubules than in the proximal tubules [179].

Numerous studies have found critical roles for HIF molecules in hypoxic adaptation of the kidneys as well as pathophysiology of various kidney diseases [177]. Given the fact HIF is the key step in renal response to hypoxia targeting HIF and its regulatory mechanisms is a plausible approach to prevent and treat hypoxic insults to kidney. In quest for novel therapeutic tools for treatment and prevention of kidney diseases, HIF-related pathways have shown promising results.

3.2. HIF in acute kidney injury

AKI is defined by rapid decline in renal function. AKI has multitude of causes. One of the most common causes of AKI is ischemia as a result of decreased renal perfusion, which leads to acute tubular necrosis (ATN) [180]. With renal ischemia several mechanisms in small arterioles will perpetuate regional hypoxia (**Figure 6**); these mechanisms include:

a. Decreased generation of nitric oxide (vasodilator) by endothelial cells [181]

b. Enhanced reactivity to endogenous mediators of vasoconstriction [182]

c. Small vessel occlusion due to activation of coagulation system interaction between the endothelium and leukocytes [183]

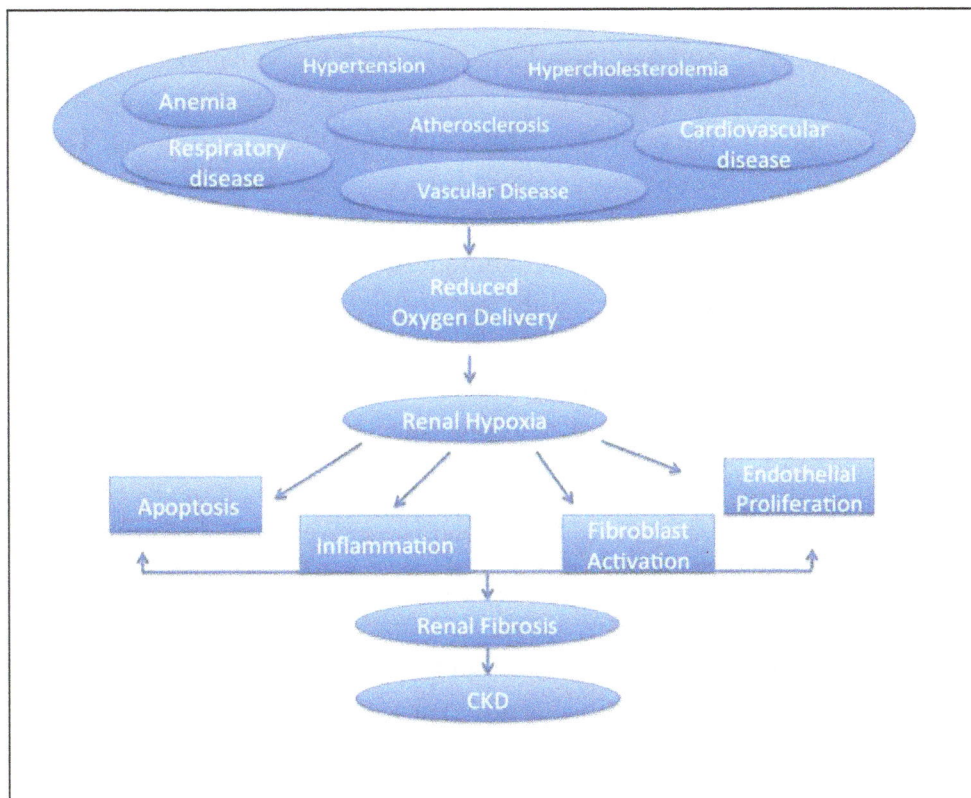

Figure 6. Diagram summarizing the interrelation between different factors causing hypoxia and CKD.

It has been shown that after renal ischemic attack, the number of capillaries in the medulla will decrease, which in turn leads to chronic ischemia, fibrosis, and progression to CKD [184]. Therefore, AKI is a risk factor for development of CKD. At the same time, patients with CKD have more incidence of AKI. In fact the most important risk factor of AKI is CKD [185]. AKI carries high risk of mortality; among patients older than 66 years with a first AKI hospitaliza-tion, the in-hospital mortality rate in 2013 was up to 14.4% (2015 USRDS Annual Data Report). Mortality rate in patients with AKI admitted to intensive care unit may surpass 50%. These data obviated the need for finding new therapies in AKI focused on renal hypoxia.

The key hypoxic intermediates mostly studied in animal models of AKI are HIF-1 and HIF-2. Rosenberger et al. showed that upregulation of HIF-1α occurs up to 7 days following ligation of a branch of the renal artery. HIF-2α expression has also been noted but to a lesser degree than HIF-1α and was confined to resident and infiltrating peritubular cells in the cortex [186]. Numerous studies have shown the involvement of HIF proteins in protection against acute renal injury [177]. Induction of HIF-1 or its target genes have shown to reduce injury secondary to various types of acute renal insult [187, 188].

3.2.1. HIF in contrast-induced nephropathy

The exact mechanism of contrast-induced nephropathy (CIN) remains elusive. Among possible mechanisms are renal vasoconstriction and decreased vasodilatation, which leads to tubular hypoxemia, decreased mitochondrial function and generation of reactive oxygen species (ROS), increased prostaglandins, decreased NO levels, and increased oxygen consumption due to osmotic demand of contrast media on tubular Na/K ATPase, all of which lead to medullary cell damage [189, 190]. Clearly, a direct link with hypoxia and CIN exists. Reversible renal vasoconstriction has been demonstrated in animal studies [191]. In an animal study, Rosenberger et al. induced renal hypoxia by a combination of COX inhibition, radio-contrast material, and blockade of nitric oxide synthase. In this study generalized HIF induction (tubules, interstitium, and endothelial cells) initiated within minutes of regional renal hypoxia. They showed medullary thick ascending limb (TAL) of Henle had less HIF expression, which may explain the higher susceptibility of this region to hypoxia [175]. These findings render regional hypoxia a plausible cause for CIN pathophysiology and a potential role for preventative HIF induction therapy in this condition.

3.2.2. Ischemic acute kidney injury

Ischemic injury in thick ascending limb of Henle is believed to play a pivotal role in pathogenesis of AKI due to regional renal low oxygen tension. Activation of HIF-1 has shown to be protective in models of ischemia-reperfusion injury. Schley and his colleagues showed that deletion of the von Hippel-Lindau (*VHL*) protein in thick ascending limb (TAL) of Henle preserved its function following ischemia-reperfusion. Notably, this study demonstrated better recovery in *VHL*-knocked-out animals by showing higher number of proliferating cells [192]. Furthermore, preconditional activation of HIF-1 via carbon monoxide or PHD1 inhibitor has shown to ameliorate the degree of renal ischemic damage in rat models of ischemia-reperfusion injury [188]. Others have shown activation of HIF-1 via cobalt chloride leads to reduction of tubulointerstitial damage secondary to acute renal injury in rats [187].

3.3. HIF in chronic kidney disease (CKD)

Chronic renal hypoxia causes apoptosis and also differentiation of tubular cells to myofibroblasts. Under hypoxic condition renal fibroblasts will also get activated. These together will lead to progressive renal failure and eventually ESRD. Glomerulosclerosis as a result of chronic high blood pressure or high blood sugar can also cause tubular ischemia by impairing tubular perfusion.

Several pharmacological means of reducing renal hypoxia are already widely available for use in daily clinical practice. Treatment with erythropoietin (EPO)-stimulating agents has been shown to slow down the progression of CKD [193]. Renin-angiotensin system (RAS) blockade can also be protective against hypoxia. RAS blockade will improve perfusion of peritubular capillaries by decreasing tone of efferent arteriols in parent glomerulus [194]. Yu et al. studied the effect of HIF activation (via a nonselective PHD inhibitor, L-mimosine) in rats with CKD. Animals underwent subtotal nephrectomy. In this study they demonstrated HIF activation can have different (beneficial or deleterious) effects on renal tissue. It was also shown that function of remnant kidney is also dependent upon the timing of HIF activation. Early activation of HIF in CKD caused increased fibrosis (rise in mRNA of collagen type III) and inflammation, while late activation of HIF showed anti-fibrotic effects [195].

3.3.1. HIF in diabetic nephropathy

Diabetic kidney disease (diabetic nephropathy (DN)) is the leading cause of ESRD. Hyperglycemia and resultant hyperfiltration will increase renal oxygen consumption. Eighty percent of the total renal oxygen consumption is related to sodium-potassium pump in cortical proximal tubule. Diabetes causes decreased renal oxygen tension by increasing oxygen consumption. Inoue et al. by using diffusion-weighted (DW) and blood oxygen level-dependent (BOLD) MRI showed tissue hypoxia in diabetic kidneys [196]. Palm et al. also demonstrated lower parenchymal oxygen tension along with higher oxygen consumption in diabetic rats [197]. In the setting of hypoxia, paradoxically, the activity of HIF-1α seems to be decreased or altered in diabetic rat kidneys [198, 199]. Polymorphism of pro582ser in HIF-1α gene, which results in altered response of HIF-1α to low oxygen, is associated with increased incidence of diabetic nephropathy in diabetic patients [199]. It appears from this evidence that HIF-1α-protective activity in the kidney is compromised in the setting of diabetes. This is further supported by the finding that pharmacologic activation of HIF pathway decreases renal damage in diabetic rats by decreasing proteinuria, improving tubulointerstitial damage and normalizing glomerular hyperfiltration [200]. There is thus indication for the use of HIF-1–activating approaches in prevention of diabetic nephropathy.

3.4. HIF in anemia of kidney disease

HIF plays a role in anemia of CKD and ESRD. Erythropoietin is secreted from human kidneys after birth. The kidney accounts for ~90% of the total EPO production in the adult human [201]. Renal erythropoietin-producing cells are fibroblasts in peritubular capillaries in the cortex and outer medulla [202].

Kidneys are the perfect choice to be responsible for erythropoietin secretion due to their regional low oxygen tension. Any minute changes in renal oxygen tension will lead to adjustments of serum hematocrit. In subcellular level HIF binds to the EPO enhancer, the hypoxia-responsive element, and activates the transcription of EPO. Renal EPO synthesis is regulated by HIF-2 [203]. HIF-2 exerts its multipronged effect by increasing EPO production, increasing iron absorption, and also increasing maturation of erythroid progenitors in the bone marrow. Studies indicate that in ESRD patients erythropoietin concentration is below normal due to dysfunctional EPO-producing cells (not due to cell death) [204]. Erythropoietin-producing cells in renal fibrosis remain alive and preserve their plasticity: although the exact mechanism of erythropoietin production in ESRD remains elusive, it is possible plasticity of erythropoietin-producing cells plays a role when signals for HIF pathway are augmented. Pathways to stabilize or even augment HIF response will mimic the state of hypoxia, which will lead to erythropoietin production; this is considered a novel therapeutic tool in our armamentarium to treat anemia of CKD. HIF stabilizers inhibit PHDs, which will subsequently cause accumulation of HIF, and as a result erythropoietin production ensues.

In 2010 a phase 1 clinical trial revealed PHD inhibitor (FG-2216) led to increased EPO production and plasma EPO levels in patients with ESRD [205]. In a phase 2-b study of nondialysis-dependent patients with chronic kidney disease, related anemia treatment with an oral PHD inhibitor (Roxadustat) was shown to increase EPO level and correct anemia. Clinical response was independent of iron intake (oral or IV) [206].

3.5. HIF in renal transplant

As of January 2016, there are 100,791 people waiting for renal transplants in the United States. Every 14 min a patient is added to the kidney transplant waiting list. In 2012, the probability of 1-year graft survival was 92% and 97% for deceased and living donor kidney transplant recipients, respectively. The estimated US average charges for a kidney transplant in 2011 is $262,900. This data emphasizes on the need for exploring new ways to save and preserve more allografts.

In the process of renal transplantation, harvested organ is subjected to hypoxia. Hypoxia-reperfusion occurs during organ procurement, preservation, and after implantation. Ischemia-Reperfusion injury (IRI) has prognostic implications for the allograft and kidney recipient. As mentioned before HIF has been shown to be a renoprotective agent and may alter transplantation outcome.

Conde et al. found HIF-1α increases in human proximal tubular cells (in vitro) after hypoxia and also during reoxygenation period. A similar biphasic pattern was observed in IRI model in SD rats (en vivo). The en vivo part of the study proved that HIF-1α induction during reperfusion phase was required for survival of proximal tubule cells and expited recovery. Conde and his colleagues also studied human allograft biopsies (7–15 days post-transplant): HIF-1α expression was more robust in proximal tubule cells with minimal ischemic damage. Again, this finding indicate a protective role of HIF in IRI. AN interesting finding in this study was demonstration of the role of Akt/mTOR signaling in HIF-1α induction. Using rapamycin (mTOR inhibitor) during reoxygenation period prevented HIF-1α stabilization [207].

Renal ischemia-reperfusion injury is an important factor in determination of the fate of a renal allograft. Immunological response is potentiated under ischemia-reperfusion. CD4+ T cells play the main role in pathogenesis of IRI and natural killer (NK) cells are part of the immediate response to IRI. Regulatory family differentially affect the immune response to the of HIF affect allograft's during ischemia-reperfusion. While HIF-1α plays a crucial role in T-cell survival and function , HIF-2α has a protective function in T-cell mediated renal IRI [208]. In an animal study, Zhang et al. showed the role of HIF-2α in mitigating NK T-cell–mediated cytotoxicity in IRI. In this study HIF-2α and adenosine A2A receptor (adora2a) worked in concert with each other (so-called hypoxia-adenosinergic immunosuppression) to restrict NK T-cell activation [209]. This finding is of clinical importance as pharmacologic activation of HIF-2α can potentially limit allograft IRI and subsequently improve the outcome of renal transplantation.

3.6. Conclusion

The overwhelming clinical and economical impact of renal disease and the limited therapeutic options available have placed a great demand on finding additional therapeutic approaches. The evidence discussed in this section suggests a widespread role of hypoxia and HIF signaling in a range of acute and chronic renal diseases and a clear indication for HIF-targeted therapies. It appears that HIF-1 activity is protective in acute renal injury, while prolonged activity of HIF-1 may lead to worsened outcomes in CKD. The protective versus deleterious roles of HIF-1 thus complicate the use of HIF-1–targeted approaches. On the other hand, HIF-2 therapies may be more promising especially in terms of anemia of kidney disease and renal allograft rejection. In either case, additional clinical research is needed in the use and efficacy of both HIF-1 and HIF-2 therapies in prevention or treatment of various renal diseases.

Author details

Deepak Bhatia[1], Mohammad Sanaei Ardekani[2], Qiwen Shi[3] and Shahrzad Movafagh[1*]

*Address all correspondence to: smovafag@su.edu

1 Bernard J Dunn School of Pharmacy, Shenandoah University, VA, USA

2 Kidney and Hypertension Specialists, VA, USA

3 Collaborative Innovation Center of Yangtza River Delta Region Green Pharmaceuticals, Zhejiang University of Technology, Hangzhou, Zhejiang

References

[1] Alzheimer's Disease Facts and Figures, "2015 Alzheimer's Disease Facts and Figures," Alzheimer's Association, Facts and Figure, 2015. https://www.alz.org/facts/downloads/facts_figures_2015.pdf

[2] Daulatzai MA. Cerebral hypoperfusion and glucose hypometabolism: Key pathophysiological modulators promote neurodegeneration, cognitive impairment, and Alzheimer's disease. J Neurosci Res. 2016 Jun 27; PubMed PMID: 27350397.

[3] R. D. Bell, and B. V. Zlokovic, "Neurovascular mechanisms and blood-brain barrier disorder in Alzheimer's disease," *Acta Neuropathol. (Berl.)*, Vol. 118, No. 1, pp. 103–113, Jul. 2009.

[4] C. Carvalho *et al.*, "Role of mitochondrial-mediated signaling pathways in Alzheimer disease and hypoxia," *J. Bioenerg. Biomembr.*, Vol. 41, No. 5, pp. 433–440, Oct. 2009.

[5] N. Gertsik, D. Chiu, and Y. M. Li, "Complex regulation of γ-secretase: from obligatory to modulatory subunits," *Front. Aging Neurosci.*, Vol. 6, p. 342, 2014.

[6]   I. F. Smith, J. P. Boyle, K. N. Green, H. A. Pearson, and C. Peers, "Hypoxic remodelling of Ca^{2+} mobilization in type I cortical astrocytes: involvement of ROS and pro-amyloidogenic APP processing," *J. Neurochem.*, Vol. 88, No. 4, pp. 869–877, Feb. 2004.

[7]   L. Fisk, N. N. Nalivaeva, J. P. Boyle, C. S. Peers, and A. J. Turner, "Effects of hypoxia and oxidative stress on expression of neprilysin in human neuroblastoma cells and rat cortical neurones and astrocytes," *Neurochem. Res.*, Vol. 32, No. 10, pp. 1741–1748, Oct. 2007.

[8]   L. Gao, S. Tian, H. Gao, and Y. Xu, "Hypoxia increases Aβ-induced tau phosphorylation by calpain and promotes behavioral consequences in AD transgenic mice," *J. Mol. Neurosci. MN*, Vol. 51, No. 1, pp. 138–147, Sep. 2013.

[9]   C. E. Zhang, X. Yang, L. Li, X. Sui, Q. Tian, W. Wei, J. Wang, and G. Liu, "Hypoxia-induced tau phosphorylation and memory deficit in rats," *Neurodegener Dis.*, Vol. 14, No. 3, pp. 107–116, Nov. 2014.

[10] G. Basurto-Islas, I. Grundke-Iqbal, Y. C. Tung, F. Liu, and K. Iqbal, "Activation of asparaginyl endopeptidase leads to Tau hyperphosphorylation in Alzheimer disease," *J. Biol. Chem.*, Vol. 288, No. 24, pp. 17495–17507, Jun. 2013.

[11] P. Srivanitchapoom, S. Pandey, and M. Hallett, "Drooling in Parkinson's disease: a review," *Parkinsonism Relat. Disord.*, Vol. 20, No. 11, pp. 1109–1118, Nov. 2014.

[12] T. Chen *et al.*, "δ-Opioid receptor activation reduces α-synuclein overexpression and oligomer formation induced by MPP(+) and/or hypoxia," *Exp. Neurol.*, Vol. 255, pp. 127–136, May 2014.

[13] C. Vilariño-Güell *et al.*, "ATP13A2 variability in Parkinson disease," *Hum. Mutat.*, Vol. 30, No. 3, pp. 406–410, Mar. 2009.

[14] Q. Xu *et al.*, "Hypoxia regulation of ATP13A2 (PARK9) gene transcription," *J. Neurochem.*, Vol. 122, No. 2, pp. 251–259, Jul. 2012.

[15] F. Shephard, O. Greville-Heygate, S. Liddell, R. Emes, and L. Chakrabarti, "Analysis of mitochondrial haemoglobin in Parkinson's disease brain," *Mitochondrion*, Vol. 29, pp. 45–52, Jul. 2016.

[16] H. Onodera, S. Okabe, Y. Kikuchi, T. Tsuda, and Y. Itoyama, "Impaired chemosensitivity and perception of dyspnoea in Parkinson's disease," *Lancet Lond. Engl.*, Vol. 356, No. 9231, pp. 739–740, Aug. 2000.

[17] S. Zarei *et al.*, "A comprehensive review of amyotrophic lateral sclerosis," *Surg. Neurol. Int.*, Vol. 6, p. 171, Nov. 2015.

[18] N. Vanacore, P. Cocco, D. Fadda, and M. Dosemeci, "Job strain, hypoxia and risk of amyotrophic lateral sclerosis: results from a death certificate study," *Amyotroph. Lateral Scler. Off. Publ. World Fed. Neurol. Res. Group Mot. Neuron Dis.*, Vol. 11, No. 5, pp. 430–434, Oct. 2010.

[19] V. Subramanian, B. Crabtree, and K. R. Acharya, "Human angiogenin is a neuroprotective factor and amyotrophic lateral sclerosis associated angiogenin variants affect neurite extension/pathfinding and survival of motor neurons," *Hum. Mol. Genet.*, Vol. 17, No. 1, pp. 130–149, Jan. 2008.

[20] S. M. Kim *et al.*, "Intermittent hypoxia can aggravate motor neuronal loss and cognitive dysfunction in ALS mice," *PloS One*, Vol. 8, No. 11, p. e81808, Nov. 2013.

[21] R. Xu *et al.*, "Linking hypoxic and oxidative insults to cell death mechanisms in models of ALS," *Brain Res.*, Vol. 1372, pp. 133–144, Feb. 2011.

[22] S. K. S. Sarada, P. Himadri, D. Ruma, S. K. Sharma, T. Pauline, and Mrinalini, "Selenium protects the hypoxia induced apoptosis in neuroblastoma cells through upregulation of Bcl-2," *Brain Res.*, Vol. 1209, pp. 29–39, May 2008.

[23] S. Li, W. Wang, C. Wang, and Y. Y. Tang, "Possible involvement of NO/NOS signaling in hippocampal amyloid-beta production induced by transient focal cerebral ischemia in aged rats," *Neurosci. Lett.*, Vol. 470, No. 2, pp. 106–110, Feb. 2010.

[24] J. Li *et al.*, "Hypoxia induces beta-amyloid in association with death of RGC-5 cells in culture," *Biochem. Biophys. Res. Commun.*, Vol. 410, No. 1, pp. 40–44, Jun. 2011.

[25] R. Perfeito, D. F. Lázaro, T. F. Outeiro, and A. C. Rego, "Linking alpha-synuclein phosphorylation to reactive oxygen species formation and mitochondrial dysfunction in SH-SY5Y cells," *Mol. Cell. Neurosci.*, Vol. 62, pp. 51–59, Sep. 2014.

[26] J. W. Błaszczyk, "Parkinson's disease and neurodegeneration: GABA-collapse hypothesis," *Front. Neurosci.*, Vol. 10, p. 269, 2016.

[27] I. F. Smith, J. P. Boyle, P. F. Vaughan, H. A. Pearson, and C. Peers, "Effects of chronic hypoxia on Ca(2+) stores and capacitative Ca(2+) entry in human neuroblastoma (SH-SY5Y) cells," *J. Neurochem.*, Vol. 79, No. 4, pp. 877–884, Nov. 2001.

[28] I. F. Smith, L. D. Plant, J. P. Boyle, R. A. Skinner, H. A. Pearson, and C. Peers, "Chronic hypoxia potentiates capacitative Ca^{2+} entry in type-I cortical astrocytes," *J. Neurochem.*, Vol. 85, No. 5, pp. 1109–1116, Jun. 2003.

[29] J. L. Scragg, I. M. Fearon, J. P. Boyle, S. G. Ball, G. Varadi, and C. Peers, "Alzheimer's amyloid peptides mediate hypoxic up-regulation of L-type Ca^{2+} channels," *FASEB J. Off. Publ. Fed. Am. Soc. Exp. Biol.*, Vol. 19, No. 1, pp. 150–152, Jan. 2005.

[30] G. M. Bishop and S. R. Robinson, "Quantitative analysis of cell death and ferritin expression in response to cortical iron: implications for hypoxia-ischemia and stroke," *Brain Res.*, Vol. 907, No. 1–2, pp. 175–187, Jul. 2001.

[31] Y. Qi, T. M. Jamindar, and G. Dawson, "Hypoxia alters iron homeostasis and induces ferritin synthesis in oligodendrocytes," *J. Neurochem.*, Vol. 64, No. 6, pp. 2458–2464, Jun. 1995.

[32] P. W. Mantyh *et al.*, "Aluminum, iron, and zinc ions promote aggregation of physiological concentrations of beta-amyloid peptide," *J. Neurochem.*, Vol. 61, No. 3, pp. 1171–1174, Sep. 1993.

[33] M. Nakamura *et al.*, "Three histidine residues of amyloid-beta peptide control the redox activity of copper and iron," *Biochemistry (Mosc.)*, Vol. 46, No. 44, pp. 12737–12743, Nov. 2007.

[34] A. Yamamoto *et al.*, "Iron (III) induces aggregation of hyperphosphorylated tau and its reduction to iron (II) reverses the aggregation: implications in the formation of neurofibrillary tangles of Alzheimer's disease," *J. Neurochem.*, Vol. 82, No. 5, pp. 1137–1147, Sep. 2002.

[35] P. Dusek, P. M. Roos, T. Litwin, S. A. Schneider, T. P. Flaten, and J. Aaseth, "The neurotoxicity of iron, copper and manganese in Parkinson's and Wilson's diseases," *J. Trace Elem. Med. Biol. Organ Soc. Miner. Trace Elem. GMS*, Vol. 31, pp. 193–203, 2015.

[36] L. D. Lukyanova, E. L. Germanova, T. A. Tsybina, and G. N. Chernobaeva, "Energotropic effect of succinate-containing derivatives of 3-hydroxypyridine," *Bull. Exp. Biol. Med.*, Vol. 148, No. 4, pp. 587–591, Oct. 2009.

[37] L. D. Lukyanova and Y. I. Kirova, "Mitochondria-controlled signaling mechanisms of brain protection in hypoxia," *Front. Neurosci.*, Vol. 9, p. 320, 2015.

[38] K. L. H. Carpenter, I. Jalloh, and P. J. Hutchinson, "Glycolysis and the significance of lactate in traumatic brain injury," *Front. Neurosci.*, Vol. 9, pp. 112, 2015.

[39] S. Takahashi, T. Iizumi, K. Mashima, T. Abe, and N. Suzuki, "Roles and regulation of ketogenesis in cultured astroglia and neurons under hypoxia and hypoglycemia," *ASN Neuro*, Vol. 6, No. 5, 2014.

[40] S. Melov *et al.*, "Mitochondrial oxidative stress causes hyperphosphorylation of tau," *PloS One*, Vol. 2, No. 6, p. e536, 2007.

[41] S. T. Brown, J. L. Scragg, J. P. Boyle, K. Hudasek, C. Peers, and I. M. Fearon, "Hypoxic augmentation of Ca^{2+} channel currents requires a functional electron transport chain," *J. Biol. Chem.*, Vol. 280, No. 23, pp. 21706–21712, Jun. 2005.

[42] A. H. V. Schapira, "Mitochondria in the aetiology and pathogenesis of Parkinson's disease," *Lancet Neurol.*, Vol. 7, No. 1, pp. 97–109, Jan. 2008.

[43] P. Khurana, Q. M. Ashraf, O. P. Mishra, and M. Delivoria-Papadopoulos, "Effect of hypoxia on caspase-3, -8, and -9 activity and expression in the cerebral cortex of newborn piglets," *Neurochem. Res.*, Vol. 27, No. 9, pp. 931–938, Sep. 2002.

[44] J. Sebastià *et al.*, "Angiogenin protects motoneurons against hypoxic injury," *Cell Death Differ.*, Vol. 16, No. 9, pp. 1238–1247, Sep. 2009.

[45] S. Mandel, O. Weinreb, T. Amit, and M. B. H. Youdim, "Mechanism of neuroprotective action of the anti-Parkinson drug rasagiline and its derivatives," *Brain Res. Brain Res. Rev.*, Vol. 48, No. 2, pp. 379–387, Apr. 2005.

[46] C. Pan, Z. Xu, Y. Dong, Y. Zhang, J. Zhang, S. McAuliffe, Y. Yue, T. Li, and Z. Xie, "The potential dual effects of anesthetic isoflurane on hypoxia-induced caspase-3 activation and increases in β-site amyloid precursor protein-cleaving enzyme levels," *Anesth. Analg.*, Vol. 113, No. 1, pp. 145–152, Jul. 2011.

[47] G. Mukandala, R. Tynan, S. Lanigan, and J. J. O'Connor, "The effects of hypoxia and inflammation on synaptic signaling in the CNS," *Brain Sci.*, Vol. 6, No. 1, 2016.

[48] A. Görlach, "Control of adenosine transport by hypoxia," *Circ. Res.*, Vol. 97, No. 1, pp. 1–3, Jul. 2005.

[49] D. Boison, "Adenosine kinase, epilepsy and stroke: mechanisms and therapies," *Trends Pharmacol. Sci.*, Vol. 27, No. 12, pp. 652–658, Dec. 2006.

[50] S. J. Guzman and Z. Gerevich, "P2Y receptors in synaptic transmission and plasticity: therapeutic potential in cognitive dysfunction," *Neural Plast.*, Vol. 2016, p. 1207393, 2016.

[51] D. Moore, S. Iritani, J. Chambers, and P. Emson, "Immunohistochemical localization of the P2Y1 purinergic receptor in Alzheimer's disease," *Neuroreport*, Vol. 11, No. 17, pp. 3799–3803, Nov. 2000.

[52] A. Delekate, M. Füchtemeier, T. Schumacher, C. Ulbrich, M. Foddis, and G. C. Petzold, "Metabotropic P2Y1 receptor signalling mediates astrocytic hyperactivity *in vivo* in an Alzheimer's disease mouse model," *Nat. Commun.*, Vol. 5, p. 5422, 2014.

[53] M. Xu, and H. Zhang, "Death and survival of neuronal and astrocytic cells in ischemic brain injury: a role of autophagy," *Acta Pharmacol. Sin.*, Vol. 32, No. 9, pp. 1089–1099, Sep. 2011.

[54] F. Adhami *et al.*, "Cerebral ischemia-hypoxia induces intravascular coagulation and autophagy," *Am. J. Pathol.*, Vol. 169, No. 2, pp. 566–583, Aug. 2006.

[55] A. P. Qin *et al.*, "Autophagy was activated in injured astrocytes and mildly decreased cell survival following glucose and oxygen deprivation and focal cerebral ischemia," *Autophagy*, Vol. 6, No. 6, pp. 738–753, Aug. 2010.

[56] Z. Liu *et al.*, "The ambiguous relationship of oxidative stress, tau hyperphosphorylation, and autophagy dysfunction in Alzheimer's disease," *Oxid. Med. Cell. Longev.*, Vol. 2015, p. 352723, 2015.

[57] T. Hamano *et al.*, "Autophagic-lysosomal perturbation enhances tau aggregation in transfectants with induced wild-type tau expression," *Eur. J. Neurosci.*, Vol. 27, No. 5, pp. 1119–1130, Mar. 2008.

[58] D. Heras-Sandoval, J. M. Pérez-Rojas, J. Hernández-Damián, and J. Pedraza-Chaverri, "The role of PI3K/AKT/mTOR pathway in the modulation of autophagy and the clearance of protein aggregates in neurodegeneration," *Cell. Signal.*, Vol. 26, No. 12, pp. 2694–2701, Dec. 2014.

[59] E. Janda, C. Isidoro, C. Carresi, and V. Mollace, "Defective autophagy in Parkinson's disease: role of oxidative stress," *Mol. Neurobiol.*, Vol. 46, No. 3, pp. 639–661, Dec. 2012.

[60] E. Kesidou, R. Lagoudaki, O. Touloumi, K. N. Poulatsidou, and C. Simeonidou, "Autophagy and neurodegenerative disorders," *Neural Regen. Res.*, Vol. 8, No. 24, pp. 2275–2283, Aug. 2013.

[61] F. Madeo, T. Eisenberg, and G. Kroemer, "Autophagy for the avoidance of neurodegeneration," *Genes Dev.*, Vol. 23, No. 19, pp. 2253–2259, Oct. 2009.

[62] Q. Ke and M. Costa, "Hypoxia-inducible factor-1 (HIF-1)," *Mol. Pharmacol.*, Vol. 70, No. 5, pp. 1469–1480, Nov. 2006.

[63] S. Guo, M. Miyake, K. J. Liu, and H. Shi, "Specific inhibition of hypoxia inducible factor 1 exaggerates cell injury induced by *in vitro* ischemia through deteriorating cellular redox environment," *J. Neurochem.*, Vol. 108, No. 5, pp. 1309–1321, Mar. 2009.

[64] X. Zhang *et al.*, "Hypoxia-inducible factor 1alpha (HIF-1alpha)-mediated hypoxia increases BACE1 expression and beta-amyloid generation," *J. Biol. Chem.*, Vol. 282, No. 15, pp. 10873–10880, Apr. 2007.

[65] P. O. Schnell, M. L. Ignacak, A. L. Bauer, J. B. Striet, W. R. Paulding, and M. F. Czyzyk-Krzeska, "Regulation of tyrosine hydroxylase promoter activity by the von Hippel-Lindau tumor suppressor protein and hypoxia-inducible transcription factors," *J. Neurochem.*, Vol. 85, No. 2, pp. 483–491, Apr. 2003.

[66] O. Weinreb, S. Mandel, M. B. H. Youdim, and T. Amit, "Targeting dysregulation of brain iron homeostasis in Parkinson's disease by iron chelators," *Free Radic. Biol. Med.*, Vol. 62, pp. 52–64, Sep. 2013.

[67] F. A. Zucca *et al.*, Interactions of iron, dopamine and neuromelanin pathways in brain aging and Parkinson's disease. Prog Neurobiol. 2015 Oct 9;PubMed PMID: 26455458; NIHMSID: NIHMS729596; PubMed Central PMCID: PMC4826627.

[68] C. Guo *et al.*, "Deferoxamine-mediated up-regulation of HIF-1α prevents dopaminergic neuronal death via the activation of MAPK family proteins in MPTP-treated mice," *Exp. Neurol.*, Vol. 280, pp. 13–23, Jun. 2016.

[69] Y. Wang *et al.*, "Vascular endothelial growth factor overexpression delays neurodegeneration and prolongs survival in amyotrophic lateral sclerosis mice," *J. Neurosci. Off. J. Soc. Neurosci.*, Vol. 27, No. 2, pp. 304–307, Jan. 2007.

[70] B. Oosthuyse *et al.*, "Deletion of the hypoxia-response element in the vascular endothelial growth factor promoter causes motor neuron degeneration," *Nat. Genet.*, Vol. 28, No. 2, pp. 131–138, Jun. 2001.

[71] J. F. Grunfeld, Y. Barhum, N. Blondheim, J. M. Rabey, E. Melamed, and D. Offen, "Erythropoietin delays disease onset in an amyotrophic lateral sclerosis model," *Exp. Neurol.*, Vol. 204, No. 1, pp. 260–263, Mar. 2007.

[72] M. Y. Noh, K. A. Cho, H. Kim, S. M. Kim, and S. H. Kim, "Erythropoietin modulates the immune-inflammatory response of a SOD1(G93A) transgenic mouse model of amyotrophic lateral sclerosis (ALS)," *Neurosci. Lett.*, Vol. 574, pp. 53–58, Jun. 2014.

[73] D. Devos *et al.*, "Low levels of the vascular endothelial growth factor in CSF from early ALS patients," *Neurology*, Vol. 62, No. 11, pp. 2127–2129, Jun. 2004.

[74] C. Moreau *et al.*, "Paradoxical response of VEGF expression to hypoxia in CSF of patients with ALS," *J. Neurol. Neurosurg. Psychiatry*, Vol. 77, No. 2, pp. 255–257, Feb. 2006.

[75] Y. Nagara *et al.*, "Impaired cytoplasmic-nuclear transport of hypoxia-inducible factor-1α in amyotrophic lateral sclerosis," *Brain Pathol. Zurich Switz.*, Vol. 23, No. 5, pp. 534–546, Sep. 2013.

[76] K. Sato *et al.*, "Impaired response of hypoxic sensor protein HIF-1α and its downstream proteins in the spinal motor neurons of ALS model mice," *Brain Res.*, Vol. 1473, pp. 55–62, Sep. 2012.

[77] L. Kupershmidt, O. Weinreb, T. Amit, S. Mandel, M. T. Carri, and M. B. H. Youdim, "Neuroprotective and neuritogenic activities of novel multimodal iron-chelating drugs in motor-neuron-like NSC-34 cells and transgenic mouse model of amyotrophic lateral sclerosis," *FASEB J. Off. Publ. Fed. Am. Soc. Exp. Biol.*, Vol. 23, No. 11, pp. 3766–3779, Nov. 2009.

[78] M. B. H. Youdim, "M30, a brain permeable multitarget neurorestorative drug in post nigrostriatal dopamine neuron lesion of parkinsonism animal models," *Parkinsonism Relat. Disord.*, Vol. 18 Suppl. 1, pp. S151–S154, Jan. 2012.

[79] D. Mechlovich, T. Amit, O. Bar-Am, S. Mandel, M. B. H. Youdim, and O. Weinreb, "The novel multi-target iron chelator, M30 modulates HIF-1α-related glycolytic genes and insulin signaling pathway in the frontal cortex of APP/PS1 Alzheimer's disease mice," *Curr. Alzheimer Res.*, Vol. 11, No. 2, pp. 119–127, Feb. 2014.

[80] N. G. Bazan, R. Palacios-Pelaez, and W. J. Lukiw, "Hypoxia signaling to genes: significance in Alzheimer's disease," *Mol. Neurobiol.*, Vol. 26, No. 2–3, pp. 283–298, Dec. 2002.

[81] M. P. Mattson and S. Camandola, "NF-kappaB in neuronal plasticity and neurodegenerative disorders," *J. Clin. Invest.*, Vol. 107, No. 3, pp. 247–254, Feb. 2001.

[82] Q. Shi and G. E. Gibson, "Oxidative stress and transcriptional regulation in Alzheimer disease," *Alzheimer Dis. Assoc. Disord.*, Vol. 21, No. 4, pp. 276–291, Dec. 2007.

[83] H. Liu *et al.*, "Sodium hydrosulfide attenuates beta-amyloid-induced cognitive deficits and neuroinflammation via modulation of MAPK/NF-κB pathway in rats," *Curr. Alzheimer Res.*, Vol. 12, No. 7, pp. 673–683, 2015.

[84] C. H. Nijboer, C. J. Heijnen, F. Groenendaal, M. J. May, F. van Bel, and A. Kavelaars, "A dual role of the NF-kappaB pathway in neonatal hypoxic-ischemic brain damage," *Stroke J. Cereb. Circ.*, Vol. 39, No. 9, pp. 2578–2586, Sep. 2008.

[85] M. Srinivasan and D. K. Lahiri, "Significance of NF-κB as a pivotal therapeutic target in the neurodegenerative pathologies of Alzheimer's disease and multiple sclerosis," *Expert Opin. Ther. Targets*, Vol. 19, No. 4, pp. 471–487, Apr. 2015.

[86] E. L. Pagé *et al.*, "Induction of hypoxia-inducible factor-1alpha by transcriptional and translational mechanisms," *J. Biol. Chem.*, Vol. 277, No. 50, pp. 48403–48409, Dec. 2002.

[87] A. Görlach and S. Bonello, "The cross-talk between NF-kappaB and HIF-1: further evidence for a significant liaison," *Biochem. J.*, Vol. 412, No. 3, pp. e17–e19, Jun. 2008.

[88] B. Kaltschmidt, M. Uherek, B. Volk, P. A. Baeuerle, and C. Kaltschmidt, "Transcription factor NF-kappaB is activated in primary neurons by amyloid beta peptides and in neurons surrounding early plaques from patients with Alzheimer disease," *Proc. Natl. Acad. Sci. U. S. A.*, Vol. 94, No. 6, pp. 2642–2647, Mar. 1997.

[89] S. Shi *et al.*, "Gx-50 reduces β-amyloid-induced TNF-α, IL-1β, NO, and PGE2 expression and inhibits NF-κB signaling in a mouse model of Alzheimer's disease," *Eur. J. Immunol.*, Vol. 46, No. 3, pp. 665–676, Mar. 2016.

[90] S. Hunot *et al.*, "Nuclear translocation of NF-kappaB is increased in dopaminergic neurons of patients with Parkinson disease," *Proc. Natl. Acad. Sci. U. S. A.*, Vol. 94, No. 14, pp. 7531–7536, Jul. 1997.

[91] J. A. Lee *et al.*, "A novel compound VSC2 has anti-inflammatory and antioxidant properties in microglia and in Parkinson's disease animal model," *Br. J. Pharmacol.*, Vol. 172, No. 4, pp. 1087–1100, Feb. 2015.

[92] A. E. Frakes *et al.*, "Microglia induce motor neuron death via the classical NF-κB pathway in amyotrophic lateral sclerosis," *Neuron*, Vol. 81, No. 5, pp. 1009–1023, Mar. 2014.

[93] J. W. Kaspar, S. K. Niture, and A. K. Jaiswal, "Nrf2:INrf2 (Keap1) signaling in oxidative stress," *Free Radic. Biol. Med.*, Vol. 47, No. 9, pp. 1304–1309, Nov. 2009.

[94] P. Shelton and A. K. Jaiswal, "The transcription factor NF-E2-related factor 2 (Nrf2): a protooncogene?," *FASEB J. Off. Publ. Fed. Am. Soc. Exp. Biol.*, Vol. 27, No. 2, pp. 414–423, Feb. 2013.

[95] L. Shu *et al.*, "The neuroprotection of hypoxic preconditioning on rat brain against traumatic brain injury by up-regulated transcription factor Nrf2 and HO-1 expression," *Neurosci. Lett.*, Vol. 611, pp. 74–80, Jan. 2016.

[96] H. Meng, J. Guo, H. Wang, P. Yan, X. Niu, and J. Zhang, "Erythropoietin activates Keap1-Nrf2/ARE pathway in rat brain after ischemia," *Int. J. Neurosci.*, Vol. 124, No. 5, pp. 362–368, May 2014.

[97] Y. Zhou *et al.*, "Sulfiredoxin-1 attenuates oxidative stress via Nrf2/ARE pathway and 2-Cys Prdxs after oxygen-glucose deprivation in astrocytes," *J. Mol. Neurosci.*, Vol. 55, No. 4, pp. 941–950, Apr. 2015.

[98]   B. Sheng *et al.*, "Impaired mitochondrial biogenesis contributes to mitochondrial dysfunction in Alzheimer's disease," *J. Neurochem.*, Vol. 120, No. 3, pp. 419–429, Feb. 2012.

[99]   C. Jo, S. Gundemir, S. Pritchard, Y. N. Jin, I. Rahman, and G. V. W. Johnson, "Nrf2 reduces levels of phosphorylated tau protein by inducing autophagy adaptor protein NDP52," *Nat. Commun.*, Vol. 5, p. 3496, 2014.

[100]   I. Lastres-Becker *et al.*, "Repurposing the NRF2 activator dimethyl fumarate as therapy against synucleinopathy in Parkinson's disease," *Antioxid. Redox Signal.*, Vol. 25, No. 2, pp. 61–77, Jul. 2016.

[101]   S. Tanaka, T. Tanaka, and M. Nangaku, "Hypoxia as a key player in the AKI-to-CKD transition," *Am. J. Physiol. Ren. Physiol.*, Vol. 307, No. 11, pp. F1187–F1195, Dec. 2014.

[102]   I. Hartley *et al.*, "Long-lasting changes in DNA methylation following short-term hypoxic exposure in primary hippocampal neuronal cultures," *PloS One*, Vol. 8, No. 10, p. e77859, 2013.

[103]   Z. Wang *et al.* Hypoxia-induced down-regulation of neprilysin by histone modification in mouse primary cortical and hippocampal neurons. PLoS One. 2011 Apr 29;6(4):e19229. PubMed PMID: 21559427; PubMed Central PMCID: PMC3084787.

[104]   Q. Yang, X. Wu, J. Sun, J. Cui, and L. Li, "Epigenetic features induced by ischemia-hypoxia in cultured rat astrocytes," *Mol. Neurobiol.*, Vol. 53, No. 1, pp. 436–445, Jan. 2016.

[105]   H. Liu, H. Qiu, J. Yang, J. Ni, and W. Le, "Chronic hypoxia facilitates Alzheimer's disease through demethylation of γ-secretase by downregulating DNA methyltransferase 3b," *Alzheimers Dement. J. Alzheimers Assoc.*, Vol. 12, No. 2, pp. 130–143, Feb. 2016.

[106]   Z. Wang, X. J. Zhang, T. Li, J. Li, Y. Tang, and W. Le, "Valproic acid reduces neuritic plaque formation and improves learning deficits in APP(Swe)/PS1(A246E) transgenic mice via preventing the prenatal hypoxia-induced down-regulation of neprilysin," *CNS Neurosci. Ther.*, Vol. 20, No. 3, pp. 209–217, Mar. 2014.

[107]   H. K. Eltzschig and P. Carmeliet, "Hypoxia and inflammation," *N. Engl. J. Med.*, Vol. 364, No. 7, pp. 656–665, Feb. 2011.

[108]   C. Murdoch, M. Muthana, and C. E. Lewis, "Hypoxia regulates macrophage functions in inflammation," *J. Immunol.*, Vol. 175, No. 10, pp. 6257–6263, Nov. 2005.

[109]   S. Movafagh, S. Crook, and K. Vo, "Regulation of hypoxia-inducible factor-1a by reactive oxygen species: new developments in an old debate," *J. Cell. Biochem.*, Vol. 116, No. 5, pp. 696–703, May 2015.

[110]   B. Brüne, and J. Zhou, "Hypoxia-inducible factor-1α under the control of nitric oxide," in *Methods Enzymol.*, Vol. 435, Helmut Sies and Bernhard Brüne, Ed. Academic Press, pp. 463–478, 2007.

[111] K. B. Sandau, J. Zhou, T. Kietzmann, and B. Brüne, "Regulation of the hypoxia-inducible factor 1α by the inflammatory mediators nitric oxide and tumor necrosis factor-α in contrast to desferroxamine and phenylarsine oxide," *J. Biol. Chem.*, Vol. 276, No. 43, pp. 39805–39811, Oct. 2001.

[112] S. Inamoto *et al.*, "Angiotensin-II receptor blocker exerts cardioprotection in diabetic rats exposed to hypoxia," *Circ. J. Off. J. Jpn. Circ. Soc.*, Vol. 70, No. 6, pp. 787–792, Jun. 2006.

[113] G. Hartmann *et al.*, "High altitude increases circulating interleukin-6, interleukin-1 receptor antagonist and c-reactive protein," *Cytokine*, Vol. 12, No. 3, pp. 246–252, Mar. 2000.

[114] H. K. Eltzschig and C. D. Collard, "Vascular ischaemia and reperfusion injury," *Br. Med. Bull.*, Vol. 70, pp. 71–86, 2004.

[115] J. Kuhlicke, J. S. Frick, J. C. Morote-Garcia, P. Rosenberger, and H. K. Eltzschig, "Hypoxia inducible factor (HIF)-1 coordinates induction of toll-like receptors TLR2 and TLR6 during hypoxia," *PloS One*, Vol. 2, No. 12, Dec. 2007.

[116] B. Crifo and C. T. Taylor, "Crosstalk between toll-like receptors and hypoxia-dependent pathways in health and disease," *J. Investig. Med.*, Vol. 64, No. 2, pp. 369–375, Feb. 2016.

[117] H. K. Eltzschig *et al.*, "Endothelial catabolism of extracellular adenosine during hypoxia: the role of surface adenosine deaminase and CD26," *Blood*, Vol. 108, No. 5, pp. 1602–1610, Sep. 2006.

[118] L. F. Thompson *et al.*, "Crucial role for ecto-5'-nucleotidase (CD73) in vascular leakage during hypoxia," *J. Exp. Med.*, Vol. 200, No. 11, pp. 1395–1405, Dec. 2004.

[119] J. Zhou, J. Fandrey, J. Schümann, G. Tiegs, and B. Brüne, "NO and TNF-α released from activated macrophages stabilize HIF-1α in resting tubular LLC-PK1 cells," *Am. J. Physiol. Cell Physiol.*, Vol. 284, No. 2, pp. C439–C446, Feb. 2003.

[120] T. Cramer *et al.*, "HIF-1α is essential for myeloid cell-mediated inflammation," *Cell*, Vol. 112, No. 5, pp. 645–657, Mar. 2003.

[121] C. Peyssonnaux *et al.*, "HIF-1α expression regulates the bactericidal capacity of phagocytes," *J. Clin. Invest.*, Vol. 115, No. 7, pp. 1806–1815, Jul. 2005.

[122] J. Zhou, T. Schmid, and B. Brüne, "Tumor necrosis factor-α causes accumulation of a ubiquitinated form of hypoxia inducible factor-1α through a nuclear factor-κB-dependent pathway," *Mol. Biol. Cell*, Vol. 14, No. 6, pp. 2216–2225, Jun. 2003.

[123] D. H. Shin, S. H. Li, S. W. Yang, B. L. Lee, M. K. Lee, and J. W. Park, "Inhibitor of nuclear factor-kappaB alpha derepresses hypoxia-inducible factor-1 during moderate hypoxia by sequestering factor inhibiting hypoxia-inducible factor from hypoxia-inducible factor 1alpha," *FEBS J.*, Vol. 276, No. 13, pp. 3470–3480, Jul. 2009.

[124] J. J. Haddad, and S. C. Land, "A non-hypoxic, ROS-sensitive pathway mediates TNF-alpha-dependent regulation of HIF-1alpha," *FEBS Lett.*, Vol. 505, No. 2, pp. 269–274, Sep. 2001.

[125] J. Zhou, M. Callapina, G. J. Goodall, and B. Brüne, "Functional integrity of nuclear factor kappaB, phosphatidylinositol 3'-kinase, and mitogen-activated protein kinase signaling allows tumor necrosis factor alpha-evoked Bcl-2 expression to provoke internal ribosome entry site-dependent translation of hypoxia-inducible factor 1alpha," *Cancer Res.*, Vol. 64, No. 24, pp. 9041–9048, Dec. 2004.

[126] M. S. Hayden, A. P. West, and S. Ghosh, "NF-κB and the immune response," *Oncogene*, Vol. 25, No. 51, pp. 6758–6780, 2006.

[127] A. C. Koong, E. Y. Chen, and A. J. Giaccia, "Hypoxia causes the activation of nuclear factor κB through the phosphorylation of IκBα on tyrosine residues," *Cancer Res.*, Vol. 54, No. 6, pp. 1425–1430, Mar. 1994.

[128] N. S. Kenneth and S. Rocha, "Regulation of gene expression by hypoxia," *Biochem. J.*, Vol. 414, No. 1, pp. 19–29, Aug. 2008.

[129] A. Melvin, S. Mudie, and S. Rocha, "Mechanism of hypoxia-induced NFκB," *Cell Cycle*, Vol. 10, No. 6, pp. 879–882, Mar. 2011.

[130] A. Adhikari, M. Xu, and Z. J. Chen, "Ubiquitin-mediated activation of TAK1 and IKK," *Oncogene*, Vol. 26, No. 22, pp. 3214–3226, 2007.

[131] E. P. Cummins *et al.*, "Prolyl hydroxylase-1 negatively regulates IκB kinase-β, giving insight into hypoxia-induced NFκB activity," *Proc. Natl. Acad. Sci. U. S. A.*, Vol. 103, No. 48, pp. 18154–18159, Nov. 2006.

[132] P. van Uden, N. S. Kenneth, and S. Rocha, "Regulation of hypoxia-inducible factor-1α by NF-κB," *Biochem. J.*, Vol. 412, No. 3, pp. 477–484, Jun. 2008.

[133] R. S. BelAiba *et al.*, "Hypoxia up-regulates hypoxia-inducible factor-1α transcription by involving phosphatidylinositol 3-kinase and nuclear factor κB in pulmonary artery smooth muscle cells," *Mol. Biol. Cell*, Vol. 18, No. 12, pp. 4691–4697, Dec. 2007.

[134] C. T. Taylor and E. P. Cummins, "The role of NF-kappaB in hypoxia-induced gene expression," *Ann. N. Y. Acad. Sci.*, Vol. 1177, pp. 178–184, Oct. 2009.

[135] S. F. Fitzpatrick *et al.*, "An intact canonical NF-κB pathway is required for inflammatory gene expression in response to hypoxia," *J. Immunol. Baltim. Md 1950*, Vol. 186, No. 2, pp. 1091–1096, Jan. 2011.

[136] M. Scortegagna *et al.*, "HIF-1α regulates epithelial inflammation by cell autonomous NFκB activation and paracrine stromal remodeling," *Blood*, Vol. 111, No. 7, pp. 3343–3354, Apr. 2008.

[137] S. R. Walmsley *et al.*, "Hypoxia-induced neutrophil survival is mediated by HIF-1α-dependent NF-κB activity," *J. Exp. Med.*, Vol. 201, No. 1, pp. 105–115, Jan. 2005.

[138] C. T. Taylor, and S. P. Colgan, "Hypoxia and gastrointestinal disease," *J. Mol. Med.*, Vol. 85, No. 12, pp. 1295–1300, Nov. 2007.

[139] A. Giatromanolaki *et al.*, "Hypoxia inducible factor 1α and 2α overexpression in inflammatory bowel disease," *J. Clin. Pathol.*, Vol. 56, No. 3, pp. 209–213, Mar. 2003.

[140] A. Kapsoritakis *et al.*, "Vascular endothelial growth factor in inflammatory bowel disease," *Int. J. Colorectal Dis.*, Vol. 18, No. 5, pp. 418–422, May 2003.

[141] O. A. Hatoum, D. G. Binion, and D. D. Gutterman, "Paradox of simultaneous intestinal ischaemia and hyperaemia in inflammatory bowel disease," *Eur. J. Clin. Invest.*, Vol. 35, No. 10, pp. 599–609, Oct. 2005.

[142] J. Karhausen, G. T. Furuta, J. E. Tomaszewski, R. S. Johnson, S. P. Colgan, and V. H. Haase, "Epithelial hypoxia-inducible factor-1 is protective in murine experimental colitis," *J. Clin. Invest.*, Vol. 114, No. 8, pp. 1098–1106, Oct. 2004.

[143] D. J. Friedman *et al.*, "From the cover: CD39 deletion exacerbates experimental murine colitis and human polymorphisms increase susceptibility to inflammatory bowel disease," *Proc. Natl. Acad. Sci. U. S. A.*, Vol. 106, No. 39, pp. 16788–16793, Sep. 2009.

[144] M. E. Spehlmann and L. Eckmann, "Nuclear factor-kappa B in intestinal protection and destruction," *Curr. Opin. Gastroenterol.*, Vol. 25, No. 2, pp. 92–99, Mar. 2009.

[145] A. Wullaert, "Role of NF-κB activation in intestinal immune homeostasis," *Int. J. Med. Microbiol.*, Vol. 300, No. 1, pp. 49–56, Jan. 2010.

[146] S. Schreiber, S. Nikolaus, and J. Hampe, "Activation of nuclear factor κB in inflammatory bowel disease," *Gut*, Vol. 42, No. 4, pp. 477–484, Apr. 1998.

[147] I. Atreya, R. Atreya, and M. F. Neurath, "NF-kappaB in inflammatory bowel disease," *J. Intern. Med.*, Vol. 263, No. 6, pp. 591–596, Jun. 2008.

[148] L. W. Chen, L. Egan, Z. W. Li, F. R. Greten, M. F. Kagnoff, and M. Karin, "The two faces of IKK and NF-κB inhibition: prevention of systemic inflammation but increased local injury following intestinal ischemia-reperfusion," *Nat. Med.*, Vol. 9, No. 5, pp. 575–581, May 2003.

[149] F. R. Greten *et al.*, "IKKbeta links inflammation and tumorigenesis in a mouse model of colitis-associated cancer," *Cell*, Vol. 118, No. 3, pp. 285–296, Aug. 2004.

[150] A. Kathrani *et al.*, "Polymorphisms in the TLR4 and TLR5 gene are significantly associated with inflammatory bowel disease in German shepherd dogs," *PloS One*, Vol. 5, No. 12, p. e15740, 2010.

[151] I. Schlemminger *et al.*, "Analogues of dealanylalahopcin are inhibitors of human HIF prolyl hydroxylases," *Bioorg. Med. Chem. Lett.*, Vol. 13, No. 8, pp. 1451–1454, Apr. 2003.

[152] D. R. Mole *et al.*, "2-Oxoglutarate analogue inhibitors of HIF prolyl hydroxylase," *Bioorg. Med. Chem. Lett.*, Vol. 13, No. 16, pp. 2677–2680, Aug. 2003.

[153] E. P. Cummins *et al.*, "The hydroxylase inhibitor dimethyloxalylglycine is protective in a murine model of colitis," *Gastroenterology*, Vol. 134, No. 1, pp. 156–165, Jan. 2008.

[154] A. Robinson, S. Keely, J. Karhausen, M. E. Gerich, G. T. Furuta, and S. P. Colgan, "Mucosal protection by hypoxia-inducible factor (HIF) prolyl hydroxylase inhibition," *Gastroenterology*, Vol. 134, No. 1, pp. 145–155, Jan. 2008.

[155] M. F. Neurath, S. Pettersson, K. H. Meyer zum Büschenfelde, and W. Strober, "Local administration of antisense phosphorothioate oligonucleotides to the p65 subunit of NF-kappa B abrogates established experimental colitis in mice," *Nat. Med.*, Vol. 2, No. 9, pp. 998–1004, Sep. 1996.

[156] S. Fichtner-Feigl, I. J. Fuss, J. C. Preiss, W. Strober, and A. Kitani, "Treatment of murine Th1- and Th2-mediated inflammatory bowel disease with NF-kappa B decoy oligonucleotides," *J. Clin. Invest.*, Vol. 115, No. 11, pp. 3057–3071, Nov. 2005.

[157] S. Hua and T. H. Dias, "Hypoxia-Inducible Factor (HIF) as a Target for Novel Therapies in Rheumatoid Arthritis," Front. Pharmacol., vol. 7:184, Jun. 2016.

[158] U. Müller-Ladner, C. Ospelt, S. Gay, O. Distler, and T. Pap, "Cells of the synovium in rheumatoid arthritis. Synovial fibroblasts," *Arthritis Res. Ther.*, Vol. 9, No. 6, p. 223, 2007.

[159] Y. A. Lee *et al.*, "Synovial proliferation differentially affects hypoxia in the joint cavities of rheumatoid arthritis and osteoarthritis patients," *Clin. Rheumatol.*, Vol. 26, No. 12, pp. 2023–2029, Dec. 2007.

[160] A. Giatromanolaki *et al.*, "Upregulated hypoxia inducible factor-1α and -2α pathway in rheumatoid arthritis and osteoarthritis," *Arthritis Res. Ther.*, Vol. 5, No. 4, pp. R193–R201, 2003.

[161] J. H. Ryu *et al.*, "Hypoxia-inducible factor-2α is an essential catabolic regulator of inflammatory rheumatoid arthritis," *PLoS Biol.*, Vol. 12, No. 6, p. e1001881, Jun. 2014.

[162] M. J. del Rey *et al.*, "Human inflammatory synovial fibroblasts induce enhanced myeloid cell recruitment and angiogenesis through a hypoxia-inducible transcription factor 1α/vascular endothelial growth factor–mediated pathway in immunodeficient mice," *Arthritis Rheum.*, Vol. 60, No. 10, pp. 2926–2934, Oct. 2009.

[163] U. Fearon, M. Canavan, M. Biniecka, and D. J. Veale, "Hypoxia, mitochondrial dysfunction and synovial invasiveness in rheumatoid arthritis," *Nat. Rev. Rheumatol.*, Vol. 12, No. 7, pp. 385–397, May 2016.

[164] C. M. Quiñonez-Flores, S. A. González-Chávez, and C. Pacheco-Tena, "Hypoxia and its implications in rheumatoid arthritis," *J. Biomed. Sci.*, Vol. 23, No. 1, p. 62, 2016.

[165] Q. Q. Huang, and R. M. Pope, "Role of toll like receptors in rheumatoid arthritis," *Curr. Rheumatol. Rep.*, Vol. 11, No. 5, pp. 357–364, Oct. 2009.

[166] G. Li *et al.*, "Interleukin-17A promotes rheumatoid arthritis synoviocytes migration and invasion under hypoxia by increasing MMP2 and MMP9 expression through NF-κB/ HIF-1α pathway," *Mol. Immunol.*, Vol. 53, No. 3, pp. 227–236, Mar. 2013.

[167] G. Li *et al.*, "Anti-invasive effects of celastrol in hypoxia-induced fibroblast-like synoviocyte through suppressing of HIF-1α/CXCR4 signaling pathway," *Int. Immunopharmacol.*, Vol. 17, No. 4, pp. 1028–1036, Dec. 2013.

[168] C. Wigerup, S. Påhlman, and D. Bexell, "Therapeutic targeting of hypoxia and hypoxia-inducible factors in cancer," *Pharmacol. Ther.*, Vol. 164, pp. 152–169, Aug. 2016.

[169] M. De Bandt *et al.*, "Blockade of vascular endothelial growth factor receptor I (VEGF-RI), but not VEGF-RII, suppresses joint destruction in the K/BxN model of rheumatoid arthritis," *J. Immunol. Baltim. Md 1950*, Vol. 171, No. 9, pp. 4853–4859, Nov. 2003.

[170] H. E. Wang, P. Muntner, G. M. Chertow, and D. G. Warnock, "Acute kidney injury and mortality in hospitalized patients," *Am. J. Nephrol.*, Vol. 35, No. 4, pp. 349–355, May 2012.

[171] M. Nangaku, "Chronic hypoxia and tubulointerstitial injury: a final common pathway to end-stage renal failure," *J. Am. Soc. Nephrol. JASN*, Vol. 17, No. 1, pp. 17–25, Jan. 2006.

[172] L. G. Fine, D. Bandyopadhay, and J. T. Norman, "Is there a common mechanism for the progression of different types of renal diseases other than proteinuria? Towards the unifying theme of chronic hypoxia," *Kidney Int. Suppl.*, Vol. 75, pp. S22–S26, Apr. 2000.

[173] C. Rosenberger *et al.*, "Cellular responses to hypoxia after renal segmental infarction," *Kidney Int.*, Vol. 64, No. 3, pp. 874–886, Sep. 2003.

[174] C. J. Schofield and P. J. Ratcliffe, "Oxygen sensing by HIF hydroxylases," *Nat. Rev. Mol. Cell Biol.*, Vol. 5, No. 5, pp. 343–354, May 2004.

[175] M. Nangaku and K. U. Eckardt, "Hypoxia and the HIF system in kidney disease," *J. Mol. Med. Berl. Ger.*, Vol. 85, No. 12, pp. 1325–1330, Dec. 2007.

[176] K. U. Eckardt, W. Bernhardt, C. Willam, and M. Wiesener, "Hypoxia-inducible transcription factors and their role in renal disease," *Semin. Nephrol.*, Vol. 27, No. 3, pp. 363–372, May 2007.

[177] J. Schödel *et al.*, "HIF-prolyl hydroxylases in the rat kidney: physiologic expression patterns and regulation in acute kidney injury," *Am. J. Pathol.*, Vol. 174, No. 5, pp. 1663–1674, May 2009.

[178] K. Nash, A. Hafeez, and S. Hou, "Hospital-acquired renal insufficiency," *Am. J. Kidney Dis. Off. J. Natl. Kidney Found.*, Vol. 39, No. 5, pp. 930–936, May 2002.

[179] O. Kwon, S. M. Hong, and G. Ramesh, "Diminished NO generation by injured endothelium and loss of macula densa nNOS may contribute to sustained acute kidney injury after ischemia-reperfusion," *Am. J. Physiol. Renal Physiol.*, Vol. 296, No. 1, pp. F25–F33, Jan. 2009.

[180] J. V. Bonventre and L. Yang, "Cellular pathophysiology of ischemic acute kidney injury," *J. Clin. Invest.*, Vol. 121, No. 11, pp. 4210–4221, Nov. 2011.

[181] J. V. Bonventre, and A. Zuk, "Ischemic acute renal failure: an inflammatory disease?," *Kidney Int.*, Vol. 66, No. 2, pp. 480–485, Aug. 2004.

[182] D. P. Basile, "The endothelial cell in ischemic acute kidney injury: implications for acute and chronic function," *Kidney Int.*, Vol. 72, No. 2, pp. 151–156, Jul. 2007.

[183] L. S. Chawla, P. W. Eggers, R. A. Star, and P. L. Kimmel, "Acute kidney injury and chronic kidney disease as interconnected syndromes," *N. Engl. J. Med.*, Vol. 371, No. 1, pp. 58–66, Jul. 2014.

[184] C. Rosenberger *et al.*, "Up-regulation of HIF in experimental acute renal failure: evidence for a protective transcriptional response to hypoxia," *Kidney Int.*, Vol. 67, No. 2, pp. 531–542, Feb. 2005.

[185] M. Matsumoto *et al.*, "Induction of renoprotective gene expression by cobalt ameliorates ischemic injury of the kidney in rats," *J. Am. Soc. Nephrol.*, Vol. 14, No. 7, pp. 1825–1832, Jul. 2003.

[186] W. M. Bernhardt, *et al.*, "Preconditional activation of hypoxia-inducible factors ameliorates ischemic acute renal failure," *J. Am. Soc. Nephrol.*, Vol. 17, No. 7, pp. 1970–1978, Jul. 2006.

[187] P. C. Y. Wong, Z. Li, J. Guo, and A. Zhang, "Pathophysiology of contrast-induced nephropathy," *Int. J. Cardiol.*, Vol. 158, No. 2, pp. 186–192, Jul. 2012.

[188] P. B. Persson, P. Hansell, and P. Liss, "Pathophysiology of contrast medium-induced nephropathy," *Kidney Int.*, Vol. 68, No. 1, pp. 14–22, Jul. 2005.

[189] L. G. Cantley, K. Spokes, B. Clark, E. G. McMahon, J. Carter, and F. H. Epstein, "Role of endothelin and prostaglandins in radiocontrast-induced renal artery constriction," *Kidney Int.*, Vol. 44, No. 6, pp. 1217–1223, Dec. 1993.

[190] G. Schley *et al.*, "Hypoxia-inducible transcription factors stabilization in the thick ascending limb protects against ischemic acute kidney injury," *J. Am. Soc. Nephrol.*, Vol. 22, No. 11, pp. 2004–2015, Nov. 2011.

[191] C. Gouva, P. Nikolopoulos, J. P. A. Ioannidis, and K. C. Siamopoulos, "Treating anemia early in renal failure patients slows the decline of renal function: a randomized controlled trial," *Kidney Int.*, Vol. 66, No. 2, pp. 753–760, Aug. 2004.

[192] K. Manotham *et al.*, "Evidence of tubular hypoxia in the early phase in the remnant kidney model," *J. Am. Soc. Nephrol.*, Vol. 15, No. 5, pp. 1277–1288, May 2004.

[193] X. Yu *et al.*, "The balance of beneficial and deleterious effects of hypoxia-inducible factor activation by prolyl hydroxylase inhibitor in rat remnant kidney depends on the timing of administration," *Nephrol. Dial. Transplant. Off. Publ. Eur. Dial. Transpl. Assoc. Eur. Ren. Assoc.*, Vol. 27, No. 8, pp. 3110–3119, Aug. 2012.

[194] T. Inoue *et al.*, "Noninvasive evaluation of kidney hypoxia and fibrosis using magnetic resonance imaging," *J. Am. Soc. Nephrol. JASN*, Vol. 22, No. 8, pp. 1429–1434, Aug. 2011.

[195] F. Palm, J. Cederberg, P. Hansell, P. Liss, and P. O. Carlsson, "Reactive oxygen species cause diabetes-induced decrease in renal oxygen tension," *Diabetologia*, Vol. 46, No. 8, pp. 1153–1160, Aug. 2003.

[196] H. Thangarajah *et al.*, "The molecular basis for impaired hypoxia-induced VEGF expression in diabetic tissues," *Proc. Natl. Acad. Sci. U. S. A.*, Vol. 106, No. 32, pp. 13505–13510, Aug. 2009.

[197] H. F. Gu *et al.*, "Impact of the hypoxia-inducible factor-1 α (HIF1A) Pro582Ser polymorphism on diabetes nephropathy," *Diabetes Care*, Vol. 36, No. 2, pp. 415–421, Feb. 2013.

[198] L. Nordquist *et al.*, "Activation of hypoxia-inducible factors prevents diabetic nephropathy," *J. Am. Soc. Nephrol. JASN*, Vol. 26, No. 2, pp. 328–338, Feb. 2015.

[199] M. J. Koury, M. C. Bondurant, S. E. Graber, and S. T. Sawyer, "Erythropoietin messenger RNA levels in developing mice and transfer of 125I-erythropoietin by the placenta," *J. Clin. Invest.*, Vol. 82, No. 1, pp. 154–159, Jul. 1988.

[200] S. Yamazaki *et al.*, "A mouse model of adult-onset anaemia due to erythropoietin deficiency," *Nat. Commun.*, Vol. 4, p. 1950, 2013.

[201] Y. Solak *et al.*, "Novel masters of erythropoiesis: hypoxia inducible factors and recent advances in anemia of renal disease," *Blood Purif.*, pp. 160–167, 2016.

[202] Y. Sato and M. Yanagita, "Renal anemia: from incurable to curable," *AJP Ren. Physiol.*, Vol. 305, No. 9, pp. F1239–F1248, Nov. 2013.

[203] W. M. Bernhardt *et al.*, "Inhibition of prolyl hydroxylases increases erythropoietin production in ESRD," *J. Am. Soc. Nephrol. JASN*, Vol. 21, No. 12, pp. 2151–2156, Dec. 2010.

[204] R. Provenzano *et al.*, "Oral hypoxia-inducible factor prolyl hydroxylase inhibitor roxadustat (FG-4592) for the treatment of anemia in patients with CKD," *Clin. J. Am. Soc. Nephrol. CJASN*, Vol. 11, No. 6, pp. 982–991, Jun. 2016.

[205] E. Conde *et al.*, "Hypoxia inducible factor 1-alpha (HIF-1 alpha) is induced during reperfusion after renal ischemia and is critical for proximal tubule cell survival," *PloS One*, Vol. 7, No. 3, p. e33258, 2012.

[206] D. Lukashev *et al.*, "Cutting edge: hypoxia-inducible factor 1alpha and its activation-inducible short isoform I.1 negatively regulate functions of CD4+ and CD8+ T lymphocytes," *J. Immunol. Baltim. Md 1950*, Vol. 177, No. 8, pp. 4962–4965, Oct. 2006.

[207] J. Zhang *et al.*, "Hypoxia-inducible factor-2α limits natural killer T cell cytotoxicity in renal ischemia/reperfusion injury," *J. Am. Soc. Nephrol.*, Vol. 27, No. 1, pp. 92–106, Jan. 2016.

[208] S. M. Nabavi, S. Habtemariam, M. Daglia, N. Braidy, M. R. Loizzo, R. Tundis, and S. F. Nabavi, "Neuroprotective effects of ginkgolide B against ischemic stroke: a review of current literature," *Curr. Top. Med. Chem.*, Vol. 15, No. 21, pp. 2222–2232, 2015.

[209] M. Schwaninger, I. Inta, and O. Herrmann, "NF-kappaB signalling in cerebral ischaemia," *Biochem. Soc. Trans.*, Vol. 34, No. Pt 6, pp. 1291–1294, Dec. 2006.

4

Stage-Specific Effects of Hypoxia on Interstitial Lung Disease

Sandeep Artham and Payaningal R. Somanath

Abstract

Interstitial lung disease (ILD) comprises a group of lung diseases principally affecting the pulmonary interstitium, for example, pulmonary fibrosis. Following acute lung injury (ALI), the fate of an injured lung progressing towards either injury resolution or pulmonary fibrosis is dictated by hypoxia at various stages during the disease progression. Hypoxia that is tissue destructive at one stage of lung injury becomes beneficial at a different stage, with each hypoxic stage involving a different scheme of molecular pathways, cellular interplay and tissue remodeling. In this chapter, we provide a detailed account of hypoxia during the different stages of lung injury in ILDs, delineate the cellular and molecular mechanisms mediating tissue remodeling in the hypoxic lungs as well as the basic and clinical findings in this field with an emphasis on future therapeutics to modulate hypoxia to treat ILD.

Keywords: acute lung injury, wound resolution, hypoxia, interstitial lung disease, PAH

1. Introduction

Interstitial lung disease (ILD) comprises a group of lung diseases principally affecting the pulmonary interstitium, for example, pulmonary fibrosis [1]. An injured lung as a result of infection, inhalation of chemical, and other harmful substances either resolves over time or progresses into irreversible damage and fibrosis. Therefore, lung injury as in acute respiratory distress syndrome (ARDS), due to conditions like hypoxia can progress to interstitial lung damage or fibrosis similar to ILD-associated pulmonary fibrosis. Yet, another important pulmonary pathological condition associated with hypoxia is the pulmonary arterial hypertension (PAH) [2]. The ARDS is a devastating clinical syndrome of acute lung injury (ALI) that affects both medical and surgical patients [3]. The official definition of ARDS was first published in 1994 by

American-European Consensus conference (AECC), according to which ARDS is characterized by arterial partial pressure of oxygen to fraction of inspired oxygen [PaO2/FIO2] ≤200 mm Hg with bilateral infiltrates on frontal chest radiograph, with no evidence of left atrial hypertension. A new entity—ALI was also introduced as a condition of less severe hypoxemia [PaO2/FIO2] ≤300 mm Hg. Arterial hypoxemia that is refractory to treatment with supplemental oxygen is a characteristic feature of acute lung injury. ALI is characterized by alveolar-capillary injury, inflammation with neutrophil accumulation and release of pro-inflammatory cytokines leading to alveolar edema [3]. Patients with ALI develop hypoxia. The term ALI was eventually removed in 2011 in the updated Berlin definition of ARDS. According to Berlin definition, ARDS was classified into three mutually exclusive categories based on the degree of hypoxemia; mild (200 mm Hg < PaO2/FIO2 ≤ 300 mm Hg), moderate (100 mm Hg < PaO2/FIO2 ≤ 200 mm Hg) and severe (PaO2/FIO2 ≤ 100 mm Hg) [4]. Hypoxia may be a consequence of ALI leading to deviation in lung function and preventing repair. Hypoxia induces destructive exudative changes within the lung parenchyma, which include the following: (1) increased alveolar paracellular permeability due to hypoxia disrupted alveolar epithelial cell (AEC) cytoskeleton and tight junction (TJ) protein organization; (2) Prolonged hypoxia induces loss of stress fibers such as actin (including breakdown of spectrin), internalization of TJ protein occludin and a decrease in zona occludens-1 (ZO-1) protein levels that are associated with trans-epithelial permeability; (3) reduced efficacy of AEC to clear alveolar edema fluid as a result of decreased expression of two major proteins, the apical epithelial sodium channel (ENaC) and the basolateral Na/K-ATPase channel which are involved in transcellular sodium (Na) transport. Thus, hypoxia-mediated effects not only enhance alveolar edema but also impair alveolar edema clearance contributing to reduced alveolar gaseous exchange capacity in ALI [5].

2. Hypoxia in alveolar edema and fluid clearance in the lungs

The mechanism by which hypoxia promotes pulmonary edema is not completely understood and is still under scrutiny. Alveolar edema accumulation is a result of enhanced pulmonary vascular permeability. Vascular endothelial growth factor (VEGF) is a potent inducer of endothelial dysfunction and thus can play a crucial role in vascular permeability [6]. Since VEGF is induced in hypoxic conditions and recovery from hypoxia, its role in pulmonary vascular remodeling and enhanced alveolar edema is prominent [7]. The source of VEGF in the inflammatory milieu of lung injury includes monocytes, eosinophils and aggregated platelets. Research on hypoxia-induced VEGF expression as a cause for pathological conditions has been carried out for more than two decades now. Studies have shown that both acute and chronic hypoxia induce an upregulation in the gene expression of VEGF, and its receptors (KDR/Flk and Flt) in the animal models of prolonged hypoxia-induced pulmonary hypertension [8]. In fact, the increase in the VEGF gene expression was seen as early as 2 h upon hypoxic challenge in isolated and perfused rat lungs while chronic hypoxia resulted in greater upregulation of the VEGF receptor genes. These studies also scrutinized the mechanism by which hypoxia induces VEGF expression by examining the role of nitric oxide synthase (NOS) and hypoxia inducible factors (HIFs) as the downstream regulators [8, 9]. Studies on transcriptional regulation of VEGF by hypoxia have revealed a functional HIF-1 binding site on the rat VEGF 5′-flanking region as a possible transcriptional activator of VEGF gene by hypoxia [9]. Further studies have shown the involvement of specific regions in 3′-untranslated region (UTR) of VEGF gene in the stability of VEGF mRNA induced by hypoxia [10]. This has led to investigation of proteins that bind to this specific region to control the posttranscriptional regulation of VEGF expression. One such protein is HuR, a member of Elav-like protein family (Elav is a *Drosophila* RNA-binding protein required for neuronal differentiation). HuR was found to post-transcriptionally regulate VEGF expression by binding within four nucleotides of a canonical nonameric instability element in the VEGF AU-rich element [10]. Thus, hypoxia regulates VEGF at both transcriptional and posttranscriptional levels. Transcriptional regulation is by the hypoxia-induced transcription factor HIF-1 which activates VEGF transcription by binding to specific promoter sequences. A study exploring possible mechanisms involved in securing efficient translation of VEGF during hypoxic stress showed that internal ribosome entry site (IRES) present in the 5′-UTR of VEGF gene functions as an alternative to cap-dependent translation during such stressful conditions [11].

Becker et al. studied hypoxia-induced VEGF's role in enhancing pulmonary vascular permeability. They showed that ischemia/hypoxia-induced upregulation of VEGF mRNA and protein was associated with increased pulmonary vascular permeability [12]. Their study was also supported by several other studies which have reported an increase in vascular permeability due to exogenously administered VEGF in skin, muscle, GI tract and airways. In their study, hypoxic ischemia-enhanced VEGF expression, which was associated with increased HIF-1α protein expression and redistribution of VEGF protein to alveolar septae as demonstrated by immunohistochemical staining. This distribution of VEGF protein in the alveolar septae was further associated with increased pulmonary vascular permeability, suggesting its role in acute lung injury and alveolar edema [12]. The enhanced pulmonary vascular permeability effect of VEGF was also confirmed by another study in a sepsis-induced lung injury model, which showed that enhanced plasma VEGF level was accompanied by increased expression of vascular permeability-mediating VEGF receptor, Flt-1 and not the angiogenic-mediating receptor, Flk-1. As a result, enhanced lung edema was observed confirming the role of VEGF in causing alveolar edema [13].

Na,K-ATPase channels present in the alveolar epithelial cells play a major role in edema clearance from the alveoli [14]. Hypoxia-induced pulmonary edema also disrupts their function and inhibits edema clearance. Studies have shown that hypoxia generated reactive oxygen species (ROS) activates PKCζ (Protein Kinase C Zeta is a key regulator of critical intracellular signaling pathways induced by various extracellular stimuli), which in turn, phosphorylates the α1-subunit of Na,K-ATPase at Ser-18 site leading to its endocytosis through a clathrin-dependent mechanism and eventually to lysosomal degradation. With the loss of Na,K-ATPase, edema reabsorption is impaired and thus hypoxia not only promotes pulmonary edema but also inhibits its clearance as observed in conditions like ALI [14].

3. Hypoxia in pulmonary aquaporin's expression and edema

Aquaporins (AQPs) comprise a group of cell membrane water-transporting proteins that are involved in physiological as well as pathological fluid transport. They have been identified in the lung and are believed to play a major role in pulmonary edema [15]. AQPs can bidirectionally transport fluid across the alveolar epithelium and hence are involved in both edema formation and clearance of edema from alveoli (thus injury resolution). About 6 (AQP-1, -3, -4, -5, -8 and -9) of the 13 different AQPs are distributed in lung tissue, and it is very interesting to study how hypoxia regulates the expression of these AQPs and thus pulmonary edema formation or clearance of edema. AQPs expression could play a major role in the pathological condition of hypoxia-induced enhanced pulmonary edema and ALI [15]. Several studies have scrutinized the role of aquaporins in pulmonary edema, and the results are controversial, yet intriguing. For example, Wu et al. studied the role of AQP-1 [expressed on pulmonary endothelial cells (ECs) and alveolar type II cells] and AQP-4 (expressed throughout the airways epithelial cells) in relation to high-altitude hypoxia lung injury. They found that hypoxia-induced pulmonary edema was associated with a decreased expression of AQP-1 and no change in the expression of AQP-4 [16]. They went on to reason that hypoxia resulted in pulmonary edema as a consequence of decreased function of AQP-1, which plays a regulatory role in water clearance around the bronchi and vessels. However, the relation of AQP-1 expression and pulmonary edema, as a result of hypoxia was only correlative and the study did not use knockout models to confirm the relationship between these effects of hypoxia. On the contrary, Su et al. showed that depletion of AQP-1 does not affect isosmolar fluid clearance and had no effect on lung edema. Nevertheless, depletion of AQP-1 resulted in a 10-fold decrease in the alveolar-capillary osmotic water permeability. They concluded that depletion of AQP-1 did not have any effect on lung edema formation and resolution [17]. Several other reports have also ruled out the role of AQP-1, -4 and -5 in physiological clearance of water in the lung or the accumulation of edema in the injured lung. Another report using gene knockout mouse model of AQP5 in hypoxic conditions showed a significant increase in pulmonary edema with the loss of AQP-5 [18]. As aforementioned, a few other reports also demonstrated that upregulation and downregulation of AQPs expression is related to pulmonary edema in different kinds of lung injuries. AQP-1 has also been shown to facilitate stabilization of HIF and has been speculated that besides its role as water transporter, it could also be involved in oxygen transport [19]. Therefore, the effect of hypoxia on AQPs expression especially in the lung and its effect on pulmonary edema warrants further studies before arriving at a conclusion [16–20].

4. Hypoxia in pulmonary arterial hypertension (PAH)

Prolonged lung injury can lead to lung fibrosis as well as PAH. Hypoxia is a well-studied trigger for pulmonary vascular remodeling and PAH development [2]. In fact, hypoxia-induced PAH is an established animal model for studying the pathophysiology and therapeutic management of PAH. PAH is a refractory disease characterized by uncontrolled vascular remodeling involving enhanced proliferation and differentiation of pulmonary vascular ECs and pulmonary vascular smooth muscle cells [2]. This vascular remodeling ensues enhanced pulmonary arterial pressure (≥25 mm Hg on right heart catheterization) due to increased pulmonary vasoconstriction and increased pulmonary vascular resistance and eventually right ventricular failure [2]. Chronic hypoxia is a well-known trigger for the abovementioned events. The mechanism by which hypoxia induces PAH has been extensively studied and involves several molecular signaling pathways. Leptin, a non-glycosylated protein, synthesized and secreted by adipocytes is encoded by obese (ob) gene, which is hypoxia sensitive. HIF-1 induces the expression of ob gene in adipocytes, and clinical studies have suggested an association between plasma leptin levels and severity of PAH [21]. Results of studies scrutinizing the role of leptin signaling in hypoxia-induced PAH show that hypoxia-induced leptin expression results in pulmonary arterial smooth muscle cells (PASMCs) proliferation through ERK, STAT and AKT pathways [21]. These results were further confirmed in ob/ob mice. Obese gene knockout mice subjected to hypoxia showed an attenuated hypoxia-induced PAH that was gauged in terms of reduced right ventricular systolic pressure (RVSP) and right ventricular hypertrophy index (RVHI) when compared to wild-type (WT) mice. Thus, leptin signaling could be a potential therapeutic target to treat hypoxia-induced PAH [21]. In hypoxia-induced pulmonary hypertension, iron supplementation has been found to be beneficial [22]. A study involving human subjects in an acute model of mountain sickness has shown that iron supplementation was associated with a decrease in pulmonary arterial systolic pressure (PASP) while progressive development of iron deficiency correlated with worsening of pulmonary arterial pressure determined by echocardiography, thus suggesting a causal relationship between iron deficiency and acute hypoxic PAH [23]. Recent studies speculate that iron deficiency may worsen hypoxic pulmonary hypertension through HIFs signaling [24].

HIFs are transcription factors comprising of an O_2-sensitive α-subunit, mainly HIF-1α and HIF-2α and a constitutively expressed β-subunit which are responsible for mediating adaptive responses to hypoxia and ischemia [25]. HIF-α and HIF-β form heterodimer and induce the transcription of over 100 genes that affect cellular functions ranging from metabolism, survival, proliferation, migration and angiogenesis among several others [25]. While HIF-1α is more ubiquitously expressed, HIF-2α expression is predominant in the lung tissue [25]. Several studies have shown the mechanistic role of HIF-2α in hypoxia-induced PAH. In hypoxia-induced PAH studies, even partial deficiency of either HIF1α (HIF1$\alpha^{+/-}$) or HIF2α (HIF2$\alpha^{+/-}$), achieved using murine models, significantly decreased pulmonary arterial pressure and right ventricular hypertrophy induced by chronic hypoxia in comparison with wild-type mice that did not have any alteration in HIF1α or HIF2α expression [26]. The role of HIFs in hypoxia-induced PAH was further scrutinized and deficiency in HIFs-related beneficial effects in PAH was at least partly due to the reduced pulmonary vascular remodeling observed in these animals. Further *in vitro* analysis on PASMCs showed that HIF-1-dependent smooth muscle hypertrophy contributed to pulmonary vascular remodeling during hypoxia [26]. HIF1α is involved in hypoxia-induced PASMC depolarization, reduction in K^+ channel expression and activity and elevated intracellular calcium concentration and pH. This eventually results in altered PASMC ion homeostasis contributing to a more contractile, apoptosis resistant, proliferative and migratory phenotype [26]. Furthermore, in human PAH patients and mouse models of PAH, dysregulation of HIF pathway was reported and it has been associated with HIF-2α mutations, which was confirmed by studies where loss of one copy of HIF-2α gene was sufficient to attenuate hypoxia-induced PAH in these animal models [27]. On the other hand, HIF-2α gain of functions is associated with PAH. Studies scrutinizing the mechanism by which HIF-2α regulates hypoxic PAH have found several ways by which it mediates the hypoxic effects. In human PASMC, hypoxia increases expression of transcription factor forkhead box M1 (FoxM1), through HIF-2α, to promote PASMC proliferation [27]. Secreted matricellular protein thrombospondin-1 (TSP-1) is believed to play an important role in vascular health and disease via inhibition of vasodilation in part by limiting NO production and signaling [28]. Vascular remodeling in PAH involves the proliferation of both pulmonary artery smooth muscle cells (PASMCs) and fibroblasts apart from endothelial dysfunction. In a recent study published from our laboratory, we showed that hypoxia-induced pulmonary rarefaction and fibrosis in mice lung, and mechanistically, we found that hypoxia-induced Akt1 expression in fibroblasts was associated with enhanced TSP-1 expression resulting in fibroproliferation and fibrosis [29]. Another study has shown that hypoxia, in a HIF-2α-dependent manner, increases the expression of TSP-1 in pulmonary tissue and pulmonary artery cells which in turn contributes to enhanced endothelial permeability (mediated in part by changes in cell-cell adhesion) and accompanied by increased fibroblast and PASMC proliferation which is at least partially due to restricted adhesion of these cells in their mouse model of hypoxia-induced PAH. Also it was speculated that TSP-1 could promote hypoxic pulmonary artery contraction through enhanced TSP-1–induced endothelin-1 expression [28].

Prolyl hydroxylase domain-containing enzymes (PHDs) use molecular O_2 as a substrate to hydroxylate-specific proline residues of HIF-α which subsequently promotes HIF-α binding to von Hippel-Lindau (VHL protein) and ubiquitin E3 ligase, resulting in ubiquitination and proteasomal degradation [27]. In patients with idiopathic pulmonary fibrosis (IPF), PHD2 expression is diminished in ECs of obliterative pulmonary vessels [27]. A study using mouse model of endothelial and hematopoietic cells-specific knockdown of gene encoding PHD2 has shown that these mice spontaneously develop PAH with obliterative vascular remodeling as seen in human PAH [27]. They found that PHD2 deficiency in ECs promoted HIF-2α-mediated (and not HIF-1α) expression of CXCL12 (also known as stromal cell-derived factor 1α) that had a paracrine effect on PASMC proliferation contributing to the pathogenesis of severe PAH in this mouse model. PHD2 deficiency in ECs also promoted endothelin-1 expression that resulted in pulmonary artery-vasoconstriction. Thus, HIF-2α-mediated vascular remodeling and plexiform-like lesions formation (due to PASMC proliferation) resulted in PAH in this mouse model [27, 28]. As discussed above, prevention of PASMC apoptosis along with enhanced proliferation is an important pathological event in hypoxic PAH. Another study showed the mechanism by which hypoxia mediates this effect. In PASMCs, hypoxia induces opening of mitochondrial ATP-sensitive potassium channels (mitoK$_{ATP}$), which results in calcium-dependent increase in mitochondrial permeability or mitochondrial membrane transition (MPT). MPT eventually leads to loss of mitochondrial membrane potential (denoted by $\Delta\Psi m$), thus preventing the cytochrome C release from mitochondria and inhibition of cytochrome C–caspase 9 pathway induced PASMC apoptosis [30]. The involvement of mitoK$_{ATP}$ channels in hypoxia-induced PASMC apoptosis resistance was further confirmed by administering 5-hydroxydecanoate (5-HD), a compound that prevents opening of mitoK$_{ATP}$ channels abolishes these effects of hypoxia to a certain extent and prevents mitoK$_{ATP}$ channels opening and PASMC apoptosis. Hypoxia-induced opening of mitoK$_{ATP}$ was not only associated with prevention of PASMC apoptosis but also increased the production of H_2O_2 in mitochondria. The effect of this ROS production was an increased transcriptional activity of AP-1, which is responsible for the proliferation of PASMCs. Thus, hypoxia through mitoK$_{ATP}$ opening prevented apoptosis and enhanced proliferation of PASMCs. As discussed, apart from proliferation of PASMCs, hypoxia-induced prevention of PASMC apoptosis also plays a major role in PAH. Another mechanism involves inhibition of the mitochondrial pro-apoptotic Bax protein expression and induction of the anti-apoptotic Bcl-2 expression, thus preventing the release of mitochondrial cytochrome C into cytoplasm and eventually inhibiting cleavage of caspase 9 resulting in PASMC apoptosis [31]. Therefore, hypoxia-HIF signaling is a potential therapeutic target to treat PAH, and several in vivo studies have demonstrated this [30–32].

5. Hypoxia and alveolar epithelial-to-mesenchymal transition (EMT)

Several groups have studied the role of hypoxia in disease progression and pathogenesis of ILDs such as pulmonary fibrosis [33, 34]. Activated myofibroblasts play an important role in the production of collagen and ECM proteins during pulmonary fibrosis. The source of these myofibroblasts are numerous, which include resident stromal fibroblasts, bone marrow-derived fibroblasts, and mesenchymal transition of epithelial and ECs [33]. Epithelial-to-mesenchymal transition (EMT) is a cellular process during which epithelial cells lose many of their epithelial characteristics such as cell-cell interaction and apicobasal polarity and acquire properties typical to mesenchymal cells. EMT is driven by a cytokine, transforming growth factor-β1 (TGF-β1) and is characterized by changes in cell morphology and acquisition of mesenchymal markers including α-smooth muscle actin (α-SMA) and vimentin as well as loss of epithelial markers such as E-cadherin [33, 34]. Active TGF-β1 binds to its receptors (transmembrane serine-threonine kinase receptor I and II), which leads to a downstream activation of the transcription factor Smad, whose target genes include α-SMA and vimentin [33]. Increasing evidence over the years has highlighted the critical role of EMT in pathological conditions such as fibrosis apart from its well-known involvement in tissue development during embryogenesis. Exposure to hypoxia during ALI could promote phenotypic changes in AEC consistent with EMT. In vitro studies on rat AEC cultured on semipermeable filters showed that prolonged hypoxic exposure (1.5% O2 for up to 12 days) induced profound changes in AEC phenotype consistent with EMT including change in cell morphology, decrease in transepithelial resistance and in the expression of epithelial markers such as zona occludens (ZO-1), E-cadherin, AQP-5, TTF-1, together with an increase in mesenchymal markers such as vimentin and α-SMA. Supporting this phenotypical switch, expression of transcription factors driving EMT such as SNAIL1, ZEB1 and TWIST1 increased after 2, 24 and 48 h of hypoxia, respectively. Hypoxia also induced expression and secretion of two EMT inducers TGF-β1 and connective tissue growth factor (CTGF) [35].

Similarly, Zhou et al. investigated the effect of hypoxia on the induction of EMT in AEC. Results from this study suggest that hypoxia induces EMT in transformed human, rat and mouse AEC lines, and freshly isolated rat type II AECs [36]. They also scrutinized the mechanism by which hypoxia induces EMT in AEC and showed the involvement of hypoxia-induced mitochondrial ROS production and HIF-1α stabilization in TGF-β1 production, resulting in EMT [37]. Treatment of cells with ROS scavenger Euk-134 or using mitochondria-deficient cells prevented hypoxia-induced EMT illustrating their importance in this cellular process. Moreover, although ROS is known to stabilize HIF-1α, their results showed that normoxic stabilization of HIF-1α failed to induce α-SMA expression, suggesting that HIF alone is not sufficient to induce EMT in AEC. Their data suggest that ROS and HIF-1α stabilization are upstream of TGF-β1 production in hypoxia-induced EMT in AEC. However, TGF-β1 can also increase ROS production and HIF-1α stabilization. TGF-β1 can either directly activate NADPH (Nicotinamide adenine dinucleotide phosphate) oxidase or upregulate gene expression of Nox4 NADPH oxidase to generate ROS [38, 39]. TGF-β1 decreases mitochondrial complex IV activity resulting in disruption of mitochondrial membrane potential and ROS production [40]. TGF-β1 was reported to stabilize HIF-1α through selective inhibition of PHD2 (a HIF-1α prolyl hydroxylase) expression thus reducing HIF-1α prolyl hydroxylation leading to its stabilization [41]. Therefore, TGF-β1 and ROS/HIF may form a feedback loop to maintain a prolonged signaling cascade initiated by either ROS/HIF or TGF-β1 leading to hypoxia-induced EMT in AECs [36].

In one interesting study, investigators evaluated the possible role of tissue hypoxia in the development of fibrotic lesions in lung fibrosis [42]. In this study, they used animal models of ALI/ARDS, in which severe inflammation progresses into the early (exudative) phase of ALI and sequentially fibrosis develops as the late (fibrotic) phase of ALI. They found intriguing effects of acute versus persistent hypoxia as seen in exudative and fibrotic phases of ALI, respectively. Acute hypoxia induced de novo Surfactant Protein-D (SP-D) expression in AECs followed by stabilization of HIF-1α expression [42]. Contrastingly, persistent hypoxia-induced HIF-1α stabilization repressed SP-D expression and enhanced the mRNA levels of an EMT-driving transcription factor TWIST, but not SNAIL. This was accompanied by phenotypic switch in the AECs exposed to persistent hypoxia (72-h hypoxia for in vitro studies) as seen by decreased E-cadherin expression and enhanced vimentin expression. SP-D is mainly derived from alveolar epithelial cells and therefore loss of its expression during persistent hypoxia along with enhanced EMT transcription factor expression clearly indicates phenotypic switch of these alveolar epithelial cells to more proliferative phenotype contributing to lung fibrosis [42].

Endothelial-to-mesenchymal transition (EndMT) is similar to EMT, which is characterized by a loss of endothelial cell-cell junctions, the acquisition of migratory properties, and phenotypic switch involving loss of endothelial-specific markers such as CD31 and vascular endothelial (VE)-cadherin expression, and the acquisition of mesenchymal markers α-SMA, and vimentin [43]. EndMT also contributes to fibrosis. The role of EndMT in pulmonary fibrosis involves phenotypic switch in the pulmonary EC lining the pulmonary capillaries. Radiation-induced pulmonary fibrosis (RIPF) may involve hypoxia-mediated EndMT as an initial pathological insult leading to fibrosis [13]. Fleckenstein and colleagues have shown that radiation during thoracic radiotherapy for lung cancer induces tissue hypoxia, in part, due to enhanced oxygen consumption by Macrophages. These macrophages are activated because of radiation-induced reduction in blood perfusion in the lungs contributing to lung injury [44]. This suggests that hypoxia plays a major role in the radiation-induced lung injury. Fleckenstein et al. also reported that hypoxia is important in triggering continuous production of fibrogenic cytokines and perpetuation of late lung tissue injury [44]. However, the precise mechanism by which hypoxia affects radiation-induced fibrosis remains elusive. EndMT of the pulmonary ECs was shown as a possible consequence of radiation-induced hypoxia resulting in lung fibrosis and injury by Choi et al. [43]. They investigated the reason behind fibrotic effects of radiation in a mouse model of RIPF and in *in vitro* studies on human pulmonary ECs. Since fibrosis is a long-term event, their investigation aimed at elucidating the mechanisms behind the early damage to ECs by radiation and its link to the later observed fibrosis. Their results indicate ECs specifically expressing hypoxic marker, CA9, just prior to the substantial fibrogenesis. They went on to show that radiation-induced vascular hypoxia-triggered EndMT in vascular ECs, and in fact, this was observed prior to the onset of alveolar EMT and thus could be a trigger to EMT as well. Thus, EndMT contributed to chronic tissue fibrosis and targeting EndMT was speculated to be a potential therapeutic target to treat RIPF [43, 44].

In conclusion, current evidences suggest that the pathogenesis of human pulmonary fibrosis might involve the recruitment of fibroblasts derived from AECs through hypoxia-induced EMT as well as fibroblasts derived from pulmonary ECs through hypoxia-induced EndMT, apart from the bone marrow-derived precursors forming the fibrotic lesions. Thus, hypoxia could contribute to the formation of fibrotic lesions in the lung and hence the pathogenesis of pulmonary fibrosis (see **Figure 1**).

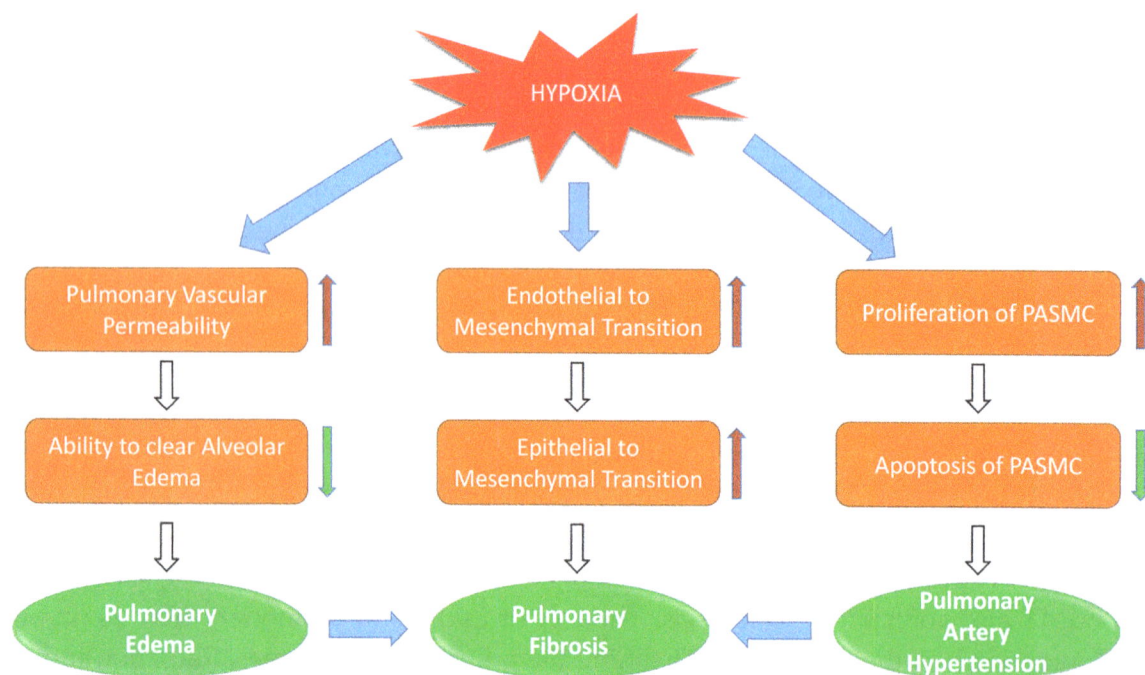

Figure 1. Summary of the effect of hypoxia on pulmonary tissue and vasculature. Hypoxia induces pulmonary edema by enhancing vascular permeability and decreasing the ability of alveolar fluid clearance. Hypoxia induces pulmonary vascular EndMT and alveolar EMT that result in myofibroblast proliferation ensuing pulmonary fibrosis. Hypoxia-induced PAH is a result of enhanced proliferation and survival of PASMCs. ALI and PAH can eventually progress to pulmonary fibrosis.

6. Hypoxia in lung injury resolution (fate of hypoxia as a consequence of pathological conditions)

While in the early stages of ALI, hypoxia plays a major role in the progression of lung injury, intriguingly in chronic pulmonary pathological conditions that ensue hypoxic milieu, and hypoxia has also been found to be involved in enhancing injury resolution. Studies indicate a protective and anti-inflammatory role of HIFs such as HIF-1α in lung protection during the early exudative phase of ALI [45–47]. As mentioned above, hypoxia inactivates PHDs and stabilizes HIF-1α [45–47]. During the acute stage of ALI, inflammation, including enhanced neutrophil activity within the alveoli, leads to an increased alveolar edema and decreased alveolar gaseous exchange capacity. HIF stabilization has been shown to have anti-inflammatory role in conditions like intestinal inflammation. The protective role of HIF activators in the treatment of inflammatory bowel disease or ischemia and reperfusion injury of several organs has been shown in several studies [48–50]. Interestingly, Eckle et al. showed the beneficial role of normoxic HIF1A stabilization in lung protection during ALI, where HIF-dependent control of alveolar-epithelial glucose metabolism function as an endogenous feedback loop to dampen lung inflammation [51]. In vivo HIF-1α increased glycolysis, lactate production and glucose flux rates in alveolar epithelium. Overall, this normoxic stabilization of HIF-1α in alveolar epithelium increased glycolytic capacity and TCA flux thus optimizing mitochondrial respiration to enhance ATP production. This HIF-dependent protection of mitochondrial function in ALI not only enhanced ATP production but also concomitantly prevented ROS accumulation and lung inflammation [51]. Hence, the role of hypoxia and subsequent HIF stabilization in reducing inflammation is prominent in resolution of ALI.

6.1. Hypoxia and adenosine signaling in lung injury resolution

Emigration of polymorphonucleated neutrophils (PMNs) through the endothelial barrier in an injured lung creates a potential for vascular fluid leakage leading to edema and decreased oxygenation [52]. The vascular endothelial adaptations to hypoxia include enhanced extracellular adenosine production during limited oxygen availability. In the vascular ECs, hypoxia induces enhanced expression of surface ectonucleotidases, CD39 that converts ATP/ADP to AMP (ectoapyrase), as well as CD73 that is involved in phosphohydrolysis of AMP to adenosine thus forming the source for extracellular adenosine production [52]. This enhanced extracellular adenosine can then signal through four different G-protein-coupled adenosine receptors, all of which are present on vascular endothelia thus enhancing adenosine signaling that is implicated in tissue protection in different models of injury including ALI. Several studies, notably couple of them from Eltzschig, H.K., et al. [52, 53], have shown the role of extracellular adenosine and its signaling in attenuating hypoxia-induced vascular leakage. They also showed that the source of ATP in hypoxic milieu is the PMNs. Hypoxia induces the production of ATP by PMNs, however, the exact mechanism by which ATP is produced still needs to be explored. This ATP is then phosphohydrolyzed as mentioned above to produce extracellular adenosine [53]. Enhanced adenosine concentrations activate adenosine receptor, (AdoRA$_{2A}$/A$_{2B}$ on ECs, which when activated increases intracellular cyclic AMP (cAMP) and activates protein kinase A (PKA) to induce resealing of the endothelial-barrier [54]. The resealing of endothelial-barrier during PMN transmigration was obviated by inhibition of cAMP formation. This resealing effect is mediated by PKA-induced phosphorylation of vasodilator-stimulated phosphoprotein, a protein responsible for changes in the geometry of actin filaments and distribution of junctional proteins as a result affecting the characteristics of junctional proteins and increasing barrier function [54]. Intriguingly, adenosine not only activates the endothelial A_{2B} receptor, but also neutrophil A_2 adenosine receptor which has been shown to play an important role in limitation and termination of PMN mediated systemic inflammatory responses. Few others have also demonstrated that PMN A_2 adenosine receptor stimulation decreased leukocyte adherence and transmigration which might contribute to attenuated vascular leak associated with leukocyte accumulation [53–55]. Thus, hypoxia-induced adenosine signaling in vascular ECs and PMNs contributes to decreased vascular leak and inflammation, both of which are beneficial in inflammatory conditions such as ALI (see **Figure 2**).

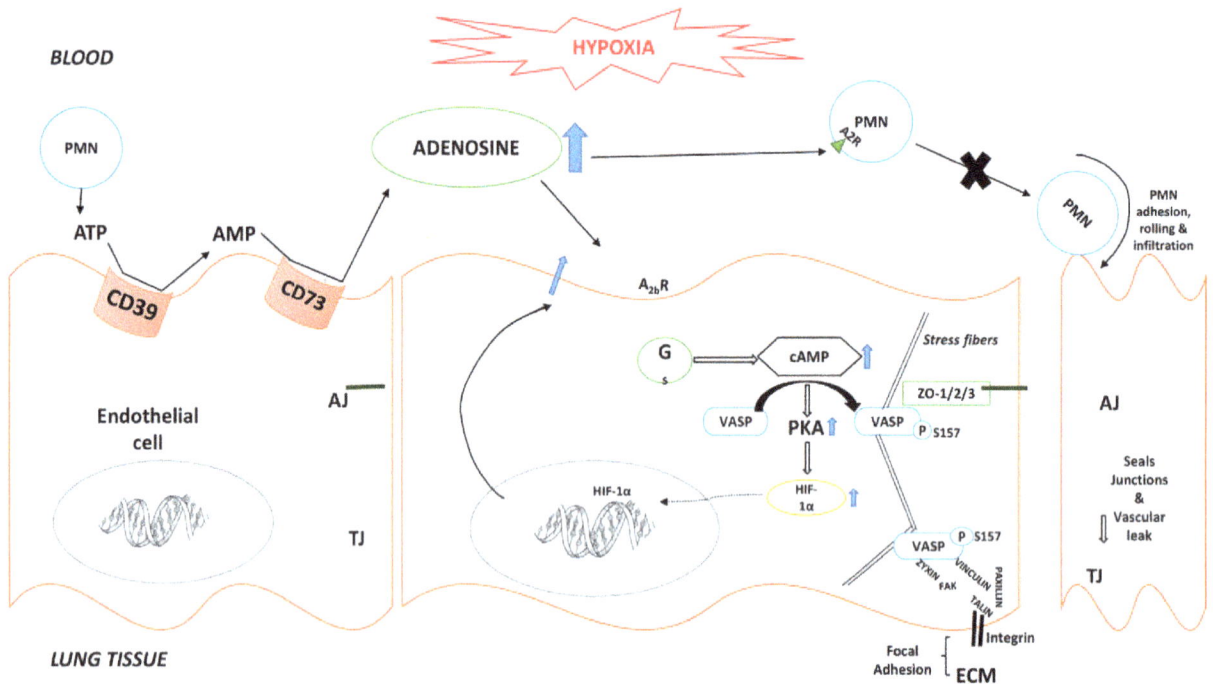

Figure 2. Hypoxia and adenosine signaling in the lungs. Hypoxia-induced extracellular adenosine production acts through adenosine receptors on ECs to enhance intracellular cAMP and PKA production. PKA catalyzes the phosphorylation of VASP, which integrates into stress fibers and helps seal the endothelial barrier by enhancing expression of AJs, TJs and also focal adhesion. PKA also enhances HIF-1A expression, which translocates into nucleus and enhances adenosine receptor transcription. Extracellular adenosine also acts on A2-receptors on PMNs and prevents their adhesion, rolling and infiltration into lung tissue. Thus, hypoxia-induced extracellular adenosine seals endothelial junctions, prevents PMN infiltration and protects lung tissue by preventing alveolar edema accumulation. PKA, protein kinase-A; PMN-polymorphonuclear neutrophils; ATP, adenosine triphosphate; AMP, adenosine monophosphate; $A_{2b}R$, adenosine 2b receptor; cAMP, cyclic AMP; VASP, vasodilator-stimulated phosphoprotein; AJ, adherent junction; TJ, tight junction and ECM, extracellular matrix.

When adenosine signaling was inhibited in transgenic mice with targeted disruption of CD73 that were subjected to hypoxia, fulminant vascular leakage, associated with severe edema and inflammation was seen [56]. Recently, studies have shown three other mechanisms by which hypoxia enhances extracellular adenosine levels, including hypoxia-mediated repression of the equilibrative nucleoside transporters (ENT-1 and ENT-2) that are responsible for adenosine transport across the membrane into the cytoplasm; HIF-1α mediated inhibition of intracellular adenosine kinase that converts intracellular adenosine to AMP and transcriptional induction of AdoRA$_{2B}$ receptor [57]. These studies indicate the protective role of adenosine signaling during hypoxia, especially in the pulmonary tissue [37]. On the other hand, chronically increased adenosine levels are detrimental as seen in pathological conditions, such as asthma and chronic obstructive pulmonary disease (COPD), and they also correlate with degree of inflammation in COPD. In order to regulate excessive adenosine signaling, chronic exposure to hypoxia eventually induces endothelial CD26 and extracellular adenosine deaminase (ADA). CD26 on EC surface acts as the ADA-complexing protein and localizes ADA accumulation on EC surface limiting extracellular adenosine accumulation during prolonged hypoxia [55].

6.2. Hypoxia and lung inflammation

Uncontrolled inflammation is one of the major players in ALI and suppression of inflammation is beneficial for injury resolution [58, 59]. Interestingly, as mentioned above, hypoxia-induced, HIF-1–mediated enhanced expression of Adenosine A$_2$ receptor on different types of immune cells, along with enhanced extracellular adenosine levels, which activate these receptors, are responsible for anti-inflammatory and tissue-protecting effects of hypoxia [58, 59]. This anti-inflammatory effect is attributed to elevated intracellular cAMP levels through activation of adenylyl cyclase. Even pharmacological immunosuppressive molecules, such as catecholamines, neuropeptides, histamine and prostaglandins are known to have their effects through elevation of cAMP levels [59]. Therefore, this extracellular adenosine serves to report excessive collateral immune damage and prevents further damage by suppressing-activated immune cells. Adenosine triggers high-affinity A$_{2A}$ adenosine receptors on activated immune cells resulting in enhanced intracellular cAMP levels to suppress these immune cells. Few studies also show that hypoxia inhibits adenosine kinase, an enzyme responsible for re-phosphorylation of adenosine to AMP, to maximize the anti-inflammatory effect [60].

6.3. Adenosine receptors in inflammation

Adenosine receptors are a family of heptahelical transmembrane G-protein-coupled purinergic receptors that are classified into four types based on the potency of agonists with respect to the intracellular production of cAMP [37]. They are A1$_,$ A$_{2A,}$ A$_{2B}$ and A3 receptors. Extracellular agonists signal through these G protein receptors and can either stimulate (Gs) or inhibit (Gi) adenylyl cyclase, an enzyme that catalyzes the formation of cAMP. Cloning experiments show that high-affinity A$_{2A}$ and low-affinity A$_{2B}$ receptors activate adenylyl cyclase (Gs) enhancing the levels of intracellular cAMP, whereas high-affinity A1 and low-affinity A3 receptors inhibit (Gi) adenylyl cyclase [37].

6.4. Hypoxia induced adenosine signaling in individual immune cells

a. *Polymorphonuclear Leukocytes (PML):* Pathological stimulation of inflammation can result in deleterious nonspecific PML bactericidal effector functions directed towards hosts' healthy tissue resulting in extensive collateral damage [54]. PMN toxic effects on microvascular endothelium are more prominent as they attach to ECs, easily because they use the same recepvtors (CR3, CD11b/CD18) that ensure PML attachment to pathogenic microorganisms [54]. Hypoxia-induced extracellular adenosine acts through adenosine receptor (high affinity A1 and A2 receptors) to mediate its anti-inflammatory effect. However, since both A1 and A2 are high affinity receptors, the overall effects of adenosine on PML might depend on the interplay between them and their expression on PML [61]. Studies show that the anti-inflammatory effects of A_{2A} receptor are to a certain extent prevented by A1 receptor, on the other hand, deleterious effects such as chemotaxis, adhesion and oxygen radical production stimulated by A1 were inhibited by A_{2A} [61, 62]. Overall, hypoxia-induced extracellular adenosine may protect the microvascular endothelium from PML by inhibiting the expression of β2-integrins and adhesion, ROS production, TNF-α production and degranulation, all of which without compromising the bactericidal function of PML such as production of bactericidal toxins and complement receptor type-3–mediated phagocytosis of bacteria [54, 63].

b. *Mononuclear phagocytes and dendritic cells:* In macrophages, activation of A1 receptor is stimulatory, while A2 receptor activation is inhibitory [54]. A_{2A} receptor activation in lipopolysaccharide (LPS)-stimulated macrophages was associated with the inhibition of IL-12 production but enhanced IL-10 secretion. In LPS-stimulated dendritic cells, adenosine enhanced A_{2A} receptor expression and intracellular cyclic AMP production along with inhibition of IL-12 production. In dendritic cells, except adenosine, other cAMP-elevating agents increase IL-10 and lower expression of MHC type II [64]. However, adenosine-mediated A_{2A} activation decreases the capacity of maturing dendritic cells to induce T-helper (Th1) polarization of native CD4+ T-lymphocytes (possible anti-inflammatory effect). Upon LPS-induced differentiation of dendritic cells, A_{2A} activation favors production of CCL17 over CXCL10 chemokines [65]. Overall, these studies suggest that extracellular adenosine stimulation of adenosine receptors on antigen-presenting cells (macrophages and dendritic cells) might play an important role in the downregulation and polarization of immune response, modulation of MHC class I and II expression, and/or decrease in IL-12 and increase in IL-10 or IL-4 production to favor the initiation of a Th2 response over a Th1 response. This effect of adenosine on innate and adoptive immune system plays a crucial role in the modulation of inflammatory response [54, 64–66].

c. *Thymocytes:* The microenvironment of thymocytes is hypoxic even under normal physiological condition when compared to other lymphoid and non-lymphoid tissues [54]. Thus, the thymic environment favors increased adenosine levels and its signaling. Patients with severe combined immunodeficiency were found to be ADA deficient (enzyme responsible for decreased adenosine levels), where ADA deficient patients had developmental defects in T- and B-cells [67, 68]. This enhanced extracellular adenosine signals through A_{2A} receptor and induces apoptosis in a subset of immature thymocytes through its cAMP elevating effects. In peripheral T-cells, activation of extracellular adenosine-mediated A_{2A} receptor inhibits TCR-triggered IL-2 receptor upregulation, thereby inhibiting T-cell proliferation [69]. Other effects of adenosine signaling in CD8+ cytotoxic T-lymphocytes include inhibition of inflammatory cytokine production, lethal hit delivery by granule exocyotosis, as well as FasL mRNA upregulation. It is interesting to note that in human blood peripheral leukocytes, more CD4+ than CD8+ T-cells express A_{2A} receptor, but on activation of T-cells increased A_{2A} receptor expression is predominantly observed in CD8+ T-cells. These studies suggest the variable expression of A_{2A} receptors on T-cell subset and how they favor the production of anti-inflammatory cytokines over inflammatory cytokines. Compared to T-lymphocytes, not much is known about the effects of A_{2A} receptor signaling in B-cell development, activation, antibody-production and class switching, and cytokine secretion [70].

However, it is very important to note that all the above mentioned effects of extracellular adenosine on immune cells were mostly observed in pharmacological experiments and is yet to be explored whether there are sufficient levels of extracellular adenosine in vivo to signal through A_{2A} receptor on immune cells. So far, there is no evidence of physiological downregulation of immune cells by extracellular adenosine in vivo. However, hypoxia-induced extracellular adenosine may have anti-inflammatory effects even in in vivo similar to in vitro studies [67, 71, 72].

7. Conclusions and future directions

Hypoxia, either as a consequence of the pathological condition during ILDs or as an etiology for ILDs has several roles in modulating the severity of the disease condition. Most of the effects of hypoxia are regulated through HIFs. Interestingly, stabilization of HIFs at various stages of lung injury can have different consequences either favoring injury resolution or worsening the condition. This complicates to provide a potential therapeutic target against HIFs to treat ILDs. Targeting hypoxia signaling was speculated to have therapeutic importance in inflammatory and ischemic conditions, such as inflammatory bowel disease, myocardial ischemic-reperfusion injury, ALI and so on. However, most of the clinical trials for drug discovery examined HIF inhibitors in the context of cancer treatment. Some of the examples include pharmacological HIF inhibitors such as dutasteride152 (ClinicalTrials.gov identifier: NCT00880672), topotecan153 (ClinicalTrials.gov identifier: NCT00117013), PX-478 (ClinicalTrials.gov identifier: NCT00522652) or digoxin13 (ClinicalTrials.gov identifier: NCT01763931) or the antisense oligonucleotide HIF inhibitor EZN-2968 (ClinicalTrials.gov identifier: NCT01120288). Apart from HIF inhibitors, HIF-stabilizing agents such as PHD inhibitors are also being studied as potential therapeutic targets in conditions where HIF stabilization is beneficial, such as, conditions which require enhanced angiogenesis (HIF activates VEGF and enhances angiogenesis) like bronchopulmonary dysplasia, a chronic disease effecting preterm neonates in which enhanced angiogenesis improves lung growth and function. Favoring the plethora of evidence from preclinical studies, in future, we can expect more clinical trials targeting PHD-HIF pathway as a potential therapy for ILDs and several other ischemic conditions.

Author details

Sandeep Artham[1] and Payaningal R. Somanath[1, 2]*

*Address all correspondence to: sshenoy@augusta.edu

1 Program in Clinical and Experimental Therapeutics, College of Pharmacy, University of Georgia and the Charlie Norwood VA Medical Center, Augusta, GA, USA

2 Department of Medicine, Vascular Biology Center and Cancer Center, Augusta University, Augusta, GA, USA

References

[1] Wallis, A. and K. Spinks, The diagnosis and management of interstitial lung diseases. BMJ, 2015. **350**: p. h2072.

[2] Archer, S.L., E.K. Weir, and M.R. Wilkins, Basic science of pulmonary arterial hypertension for clinicians: new concepts and experimental therapies. Circulation, 2010. **121**(18): p. 2045–66.

[3] Ware, L.B. and M.A. Matthay, The acute respiratory distress syndrome. N Engl J Med, 2000. **342**(18): p. 1334–49.

[4] Ranieri, V.M., et al., Acute respiratory distress syndrome: the Berlin Definition. JAMA, 2012. **307**(23): p. 2526–33.

[5] Bouvry, D., et al., Hypoxia-induced cytoskeleton disruption in alveolar epithelial cells. Am J Respir Cell Mol Biol, 2006. **35**(5): p. 519–27.

[6] Proescholdt, M.A., et al., Vascular endothelial growth factor (VEGF) modulates vascular permeability and inflammation in rat brain. J Neuropathol Exp Neurol, 1999. **58**(6): p. 613–27.

[7] Shweiki, D., et al., Vascular endothelial growth factor induced by hypoxia may mediate hypoxia-initiated angiogenesis. Nature, 1992. **359**(6398): p. 843–5.

[8] Tuder, R.M., B.E. Flook, and N.F. Voelkel, Increased gene expression for VEGF and the VEGF receptors KDR/Flk and Flt in lungs exposed to acute or to chronic hypoxia. Modulation of gene expression by nitric oxide. J Clin Invest, 1995. **95**(4): p. 1798–807.

[9] Levy, A.P., et al., Transcriptional regulation of the rat vascular endothelial growth factor gene by hypoxia. J Biol Chem, 1995. **270**(22): p. 13333–40.

[10] Levy, N.S., et al., Hypoxic stabilization of vascular endothelial growth factor mRNA by the RNA-binding protein HuR. J Biol Chem, 1998. **273**(11): p. 6417–23.

[11] Stein, I., et al., Translation of vascular endothelial growth factor mRNA by internal ribosome entry: implications for translation under hypoxia. Mol Cell Biol, 1998. **18**(6): p. 3112–9.

[12] Becker, P.M., et al., Oxygen-independent upregulation of vascular endothelial growth factor and vascular barrier dysfunction during ventilated pulmonary ischemia in isolated ferret lungs. Am J Respir Cell Mol Biol, 2000. **22**(3): p. 272–9.

[13] Jesmin, S., et al., Time-dependent alterations of VEGF and its signaling molecules in acute lung injury in a rat model of sepsis. Inflammation, 2012. **35**(2): p. 484–500.

[14] Lecuona, E., H.E. Trejo, and J.I. Sznajder, Regulation of Na,K-ATPase during acute lung injury. J Bioenerg Biomembr, 2007. **39**(5–6): p. 391–5.

[15] Borok, Z. and A.S. Verkman, Lung edema clearance: 20 years of progress: invited review: role of aquaporin water channels in fluid transport in lung and airways. J Appl Physiol (1985), 2002. **93**(6): p. 2199–206.

[16] Wu, Y., et al., Expression of aquaporin 1 and 4 in rats with acute hypoxic lung injury and its significance. Genet Mol Res, 2015. **14**(4): p. 12756–64.

[17] Su, X., et al., The role of aquaporin-1 (AQP1) expression in a murine model of lipopolysaccharide-induced acute lung injury. Respir Physiol Neurobiol, 2004. **142**(1): p. 1–11.

[18] She, J., et al., New insights of aquaporin 5 in the pathogenesis of high altitude pulmonary edema. Diagn Pathol, 2013. **8**: p. 193.

[19] Singha, O., et al., Pulmonary edema due to oral gavage in a toxicological study related to aquaporin-1, -4 and -5 expression. J Toxicol Pathol, 2013. **26**(3): p. 283–91.

[20] Echevarria, M., et al., Development of cytosolic hypoxia and hypoxia-inducible factor stabilization are facilitated by aquaporin-1 expression. J Biol Chem, 2007. **282**(41): p. 30207–15.

[21] Chai, S., et al., Leptin knockout attenuates hypoxia-induced pulmonary arterial hypertension by inhibiting proliferation of pulmonary arterial smooth muscle cells. Transl Res, 2015. **166**(6): p. 772–82.

[22] Shimoda, L.A. and G.L. Semenza, HIF and the lung: role of hypoxia-inducible factors in pulmonary development and disease. Am J Respir Crit Care Med, 2011. **183**(2): p. 152–6.

[23] Smith, T.G., et al., Effects of iron supplementation and depletion on hypoxic pulmonary hypertension: two randomized controlled trials. JAMA, 2009. **302**(13): p. 1444–50.

[24] Robinson, J.C., et al., The crossroads of iron with hypoxia and cellular metabolism. Implications in the pathobiology of pulmonary hypertension. Am J Respir Cell Mol Biol, 2014. **51**(6): p. 721–9.

[25] Brusselmans, K., et al., Heterozygous deficiency of hypoxia-inducible factor-2alpha protects mice against pulmonary hypertension and right ventricular dysfunction during prolonged hypoxia. J Clin Invest, 2003. **111**(10): p. 1519–27.

[26] Yu, A.Y., et al., Impaired physiological responses to chronic hypoxia in mice partially deficient for hypoxia-inducible factor 1alpha. J Clin Invest, 1999. **103**(5): p. 691–6.

[27] Dai, Z., et al., Prolyl-4 Hydroxylase 2 (PHD2) deficiency in endothelial cells and hematopoietic cells induces obliterative vascular remodeling and severe pulmonary arterial hypertension in mice and humans through hypoxia-inducible factor-2alpha. Circulation, 2016. **133**(24): p. 2447–58.

[28] Labrousse-Arias, D., et al., HIF-2alpha-mediated induction of pulmonary thrombospondin-1 contributes to hypoxia-driven vascular remodelling and vasoconstriction. Cardiovasc Res, 2016. **109**(1): p. 115–30.

[29] Abdalla, M., et al., The Akt inhibitor, triciribine, ameliorates chronic hypoxia-induced vascular pruning and TGFbeta-induced pulmonary fibrosis. Br J Pharmacol, 2015. **172**(16): p. 4173–88.

[30] Hu, H.L., et al., Effects of mitochondrial potassium channel and membrane potential on hypoxic human pulmonary artery smooth muscle cells. Am J Respir Cell Mol Biol, 2010. **42**(6): p. 661–6.

[31] Huang, X., et al., Salidroside attenuates chronic hypoxia-induced pulmonary hypertension via adenosine A2a receptor related mitochondria-dependent apoptosis pathway. J Mol Cell Cardiol, 2015. **82**: p. 153–66.

[32] Peng, X., et al., Involvement of calcium-sensing receptors in hypoxia-induced vascular remodeling and pulmonary hypertension by promoting phenotypic modulation of small pulmonary arteries. Mol Cell Biochem, 2014. **396**(1–2): p. 87–98.

[33] Thiery, J.P. and J.P. Sleeman, Complex networks orchestrate epithelial-mesenchymal transitions. Nat Rev Mol Cell Biol, 2006. **7**(2): p. 131–42.

[34] Zavadil, J. and E.P. Bottinger, TGF-beta and epithelial-to-mesenchymal transitions. Oncogene, 2005. **24**(37): p. 5764–74.

[35] Uzunhan, Y., et al., Mesenchymal stem cells protect from hypoxia-induced alveolar epithelial-mesenchymal transition. Am J Physiol Lung Cell Mol Physiol, 2016. **310**(5): p. L439-51.

[36] Zhou, G., et al., Hypoxia-induced alveolar epithelial-mesenchymal transition requires mitochondrial ROS and hypoxia-inducible factor 1. Am J Physiol Lung Cell Mol Physiol, 2009. **297**(6): p. L1120–30.

[37] Ohta, A. and M. Sitkovsky, Role of G-protein-coupled adenosine receptors in downregulation of inflammation and protection from tissue damage. Nature, 2001. **414**(6866): p. 916–20.

[38] Murillo, M.M., et al., Activation of NADPH oxidase by transforming growth factor-beta in hepatocytes mediates up-regulation of epidermal growth factor receptor ligands through a nuclear factor-kappaB-dependent mechanism. Biochem J, 2007. **405**(2): p. 251–9.

[39] Sturrock, A., et al., Transforming growth factor-beta1 induces Nox4 NAD(P)H oxidase and reactive oxygen species-dependent proliferation in human pulmonary artery smooth muscle cells. Am J Physiol Lung Cell Mol Physiol, 2006. **290**(4): p. L661–l673.

[40] Yoon, Y.S., et al., TGF beta1 induces prolonged mitochondrial ROS generation through decreased complex IV activity with senescent arrest in Mv1Lu cells. Oncogene, 2005. **24**(11): p. 1895–903.

[41] McMahon, S., et al., Transforming growth factor beta1 induces hypoxia-inducible factor-1 stabilization through selective inhibition of PHD2 expression. J Biol Chem, 2006. **281**(34): p. 24171–81.

[42] Sakamoto, K., et al., Differential modulation of surfactant protein D under acute and persistent hypoxia in acute lung injury. Am J Physiol Lung Cell Mol Physiol, 2012. **303**(1): p. L43–53.

[43] Choi, S.H., et al., A Hypoxia-Induced Vascular Endothelial-to-Mesenchymal Transition in Development of Radiation-Induced Pulmonary Fibrosis. Clin Cancer Res, 2015. **21**(16): p. 3716–26.

[44] Fleckenstein, K., et al., Temporal onset of hypoxia and oxidative stress after pulmonary irradiation. Int J Radiat Oncol Biol Phys, 2007. **68**(1): p. 196–204.

[45] Kaelin, W.G., Jr. and P.J. Ratcliffe, Oxygen sensing by metazoans: the central role of the HIF hydroxylase pathway. Mol Cell, 2008. **30**(4): p. 393–402.

[46] Eltzschig, H.K., D.L. Bratton, and S.P. Colgan, Targeting hypoxia signalling for the treatment of ischaemic and inflammatory diseases. Nat Rev Drug Discov, 2014. **13**(11): p. 852–69.

[47] Vohwinkel, C.U., S. Hoegl, and H.K. Eltzschig, Hypoxia signaling during acute lung injury. J Appl Physiol (1985), 2015. **119**(10): p. 1157–63.

[48] Colgan, S.P. and H.K. Eltzschig, Adenosine and hypoxia-inducible factor signaling in intestinal injury and recovery. Annu Rev Physiol, 2012. **74**: p. 153–75.

[49] Cummins, E.P., et al., The hydroxylase inhibitor dimethyloxalylglycine is protective in a murine model of colitis. Gastroenterology, 2008. **134**(1): p. 156–65.

[50] Eltzschig, H.K. and T. Eckle, Ischemia and reperfusion--from mechanism to translation. Nat Med, 2011. **17**(11): p. 1391–401.

[51] Eckle, T., et al., HIF1A reduces acute lung injury by optimizing carbohydrate metabolism in the alveolar epithelium. PLoS Biol, 2013. **11**(9): p. e1001665.

[52] Eltzschig, H.K., et al., Coordinated adenine nucleotide phosphohydrolysis and nucleoside signaling in posthypoxic endothelium: role of ectonucleotidases and adenosine A2B receptors. J Exp Med, 2003. **198**(5): p. 783–96.

[53] Eltzschig, H.K., et al., Endogenous adenosine produced during hypoxia attenuates neutrophil accumulation: coordination by extracellular nucleotide metabolism. Blood, 2004. **104**(13): p. 3986–92.

[54] Sitkovsky, M.V., et al., Physiological control of immune response and inflammatory tissue damage by hypoxia-inducible factors and adenosine A2A receptors. Annu Rev Immunol, 2004. **22**: p. 657–82.

[55] Eltzschig, H.K., et al., Endothelial catabolism of extracellular adenosine during hypoxia: the role of surface adenosine deaminase and CD26. Blood, 2006. **108**(5): p. 1602–10.

[56] Thompson, L.F., et al., Crucial role for ecto-5'-nucleotidase (CD73) in vascular leakage during hypoxia. J Exp Med, 2004. **200**(11): p. 1395–405.

[57] Morote-Garcia, J.C., et al., HIF-1-dependent repression of adenosine kinase attenuates hypoxia-induced vascular leak. Blood, 2008. **111**(12): p. 5571–80.

[58] Clambey, E.T., et al., Hypoxia-inducible factor-1 alpha-dependent induction of FoxP3 drives regulatory T-cell abundance and function during inflammatory hypoxia of the mucosa. Proc Natl Acad Sci U S A, 2012. **109**(41): p. E2784–93.

[59] Bruzzese, L., et al., NF-kappaB enhances hypoxia-driven T-cell immunosuppression via upregulation of adenosine A(2A) receptors. Cell Signal, 2014. **26**(5): p. 1060–7.

[60] Kohler, D., et al., Inhibition of Adenosine Kinase Attenuates Acute Lung Injury. Crit Care Med, 2016. **44**(4): p. e181–9.

[61] Cronstein, B.N., et al., The adenosine/neutrophil paradox resolved: human neutrophils possess both A1 and A2 receptors that promote chemotaxis and inhibit O2 generation, respectively. J Clin Invest, 1990. **85**(4): p. 1150–7.

[62] Cronstein, B.N., et al., Adenosine: an endogenous inhibitor of neutrophil-mediated injury to endothelial cells. J Clin Invest, 1986. **78**(3): p. 760–70.

[63] Thiel, M., et al., Effects of adenosine on the functions of circulating polymorphonuclear leukocytes during hyperdynamic endotoxemia. Infect Immun, 1997. **65**(6): p. 2136–44.

[64] Panther, E., et al., Expression and function of adenosine receptors in human dendritic cells. FASEB J, 2001. **15**(11): p. 1963–70.

[65] Panther, E., et al., Adenosine affects expression of membrane molecules, cytokine and chemokine release, and the T-cell stimulatory capacity of human dendritic cells. Blood, 2003. **101**(10): p. 3985–90.

[66] Xaus, J., et al., IFN-gamma up-regulates the A2B adenosine receptor expression in macrophages: a mechanism of macrophage deactivation. J Immunol, 1999. **162**(6): p. 3607–14.

[67] Apasov, S.G. and M.V. Sitkovsky, The extracellular versus intracellular mechanisms of inhibition of TCR-triggered activation in thymocytes by adenosine under conditions of inhibited adenosine deaminase. Int Immunol, 1999. **11**(2): p. 179–89.

[68] Aldrich, M.B., et al., Adenosine deaminase-deficient mice: models for the study of lymphocyte development and adenosine signaling. Adv Exp Med Biol, 2000. **486**: p. 57–63.

[69] Huang, S., et al., Role of A2a extracellular adenosine receptor-mediated signaling in adenosine-mediated inhibition of T-cell activation and expansion. Blood, 1997. **90**(4): p. 1600–10.

[70] Kojima, H., et al., Abnormal B lymphocyte development and autoimmunity in hypoxia-inducible factor 1alpha-deficient chimeric mice. Proc Natl Acad Sci U S A, 2002. **99**(4): p. 2170–4.

[71] Hale, L.P., et al., Hypoxia in the thymus: role of oxygen tension in thymocyte survival. Am J Physiol Heart Circ Physiol, 2002. **282**(4): p. H1467–77.

[72] Caldwell, C.C., et al., Differential effects of physiologically relevant hypoxic conditions on T lymphocyte development and effector functions. J Immunol, 2001. **167**(11): p. 6140–9.

5

Adaptations to Chronic Hypoxia Combined with Erythropoietin Deficiency in Cerebral and Cardiac Tissues

Raja El Hasnaoui-Saadani

Abstract

Chronic anemia-induced hypoxia triggers regulatory pathways that mediate long-term adaptive cardiac and cerebral changes, particularly at the transcriptional level. These adaptative mechanisms include a regulated cerebral blood flow and cardiac output, angiogenesis and cytoprotection triggered by hypoxia-inducible factor 1 alpha (HIF-1α), vascular endothelial growth factor (VEGF), neuronal nitric oxide synthase (nNOS) and Epo pathways. All these compensatory mechanisms aim to optimize oxygen delivery and to protect the brain and heart from hypoxic injury. We reviewed the effects of chronic hypobaric hypoxia as well as chronic anemia in the heart and brain, and we compared for the first time the effects of chronic hypobaric hypoxia combined with a severe lack of Epo (chronic anemia) in these vital organs. Functional cardiac adaptations such as cardiac hypertrophy, increased cardiac output as well as angiogenesis occurred along with the activation of HIF1α/VEGF and Epo/EpoR pathways under chronic anemia or hypoxia. Similarly, cerebrovascular adaptations take place through the same molecular mechanisms under chronic hypoxia or anemia. However, when both arterial pressure and content of oxygen are decreased, the cerebral and cardiac adaptative mechanisms showed their limitations. In addition, cerebral and cardiac cell injuries may have occurred following the combined effect of chronic anemia and hypoxia. By emphasizing the anemia and hypoxia-induced cerebral and myocardial adaptations, this review highlighted the crucial role of Epo in its non-erythropoietic functions such as angiogenesis and neuroprotection. Indeed, a better understanding of these protective mechanisms is of great clinical importance to the development of new therapeutic strategies for the management of ischemic heart and brain.

Keywords: chronic hypoxia, chronic anemia, angiogenesis, cardiac function, cerebral blood flow, oxygen homeostasis, neuroprotection, HIF-1-VEGF-Epo

1. Introduction

Inadequate level of oxygen like in chronic hypoxia or anemia is especially detrimental for cerebral and heart tissues. Indeed, hypoxia plays an important role in the pathogenesis of cerebral and myocardial ischemia, and chronic heart and lung diseases [1]. That is why specific mechanisms at a systemic, cellular and molecular level take place to maintain the oxygen homeostasis. It is important to clearly distinguish the differences between hypoxia and anemia. Hypoxia is a reduction of arterial pressure of oxygen (PaO_2), while anemia is a reduction of arterial content of oxygen (CaO_2) as it occurs during a decrease in hemoglobin concentration. This review focus mainly on chronic hypobaric hypoxia that occurs at high altitude and chronic anemia is referred to our model of transgenic mice that presents a constitutive erythropoietin deficiency. Furthermore, emphasis is placed on effects of chronic hypoxia and anemia in the cerebral and cardiac tissues. The discussion is mostly based on animal studies unless otherwise indicated, even though similarities of adaptative mechanisms are shown by human studies [2, 3].

Chronic hypoxia promotes angiogenesis by modulating the transcriptional regulator hypoxia-inducible factor 1 alpha (HIF-1α), which in turn triggers the upregulation of the erythropoietin [4], a major factor of acclimatization to hypoxia. HIF-1α is a master regulator of the hypoxic response and its proangiogenic activities include regulation of vascular endothelial growth factor (VEGF), but also Epo and its receptors (EpoR) [1, 5]. Erythropoietin primarily regulates red blood cell formation, and Epo serum levels are increased under hypoxic stress (e.g., anemia and altitude) [6]. However, several non-hematopoietic functions of Epo and its receptors have been exposed by experimental studies using genetically modified mice [7]. It is of great clinical importance that Epo has been shown to have protective functions in many different tissues. Indeed, these studies using recombinant human EPO (rHuEPO) suggested new therapeutic indications of Epo for the management of ischemic injuries of several tissues such as myocardium and brain [8–10].

Epo-induced angiogenesis may lead to an improvement in brain perfusion since Epo protects vascular bed integrity and stimulates angiogenesis [11–14] by acting indirectly on endothelial cells via activation of VEGF/VEGF receptor system, which is the most important regulator of endothelial growth and angiogenesis. Furthermore, Epo may have a positive effect on cerebral vasculature in addition to the cerebral blood flow (CBF) through alteration in nitric oxide (NO) production, which mainly derived from arginine and catalyzed by endothelial nitric oxide synthase (eNOS) [15]. Therefore, it seems that cellular protection and angiogenesis in heart and brain tissues are the dual role of erythropoietin and VEGF. These both cytokines are triggered by HIF-1α to maintain an adequate cellular oxygen supply and protect the brain and heart against hypoxic and or anemic injuries.

Our model of erythropoietin-SV40 T antigen (Epo-TAg[h]) transgenic mice has a targeted disruption in the 5′ untranslated region of the Epo gene that dramatically reduces its expression. The homozygous animals are thus severely and chronically anemic [16, 17]. Therefore, these transgenic anemic mice provided us an interesting model to study the adaptive mechanisms to chronic anemia and hypoxia, especially in vital organs, such as brain and heart. The present review aims to give a brief synthesis of adaptations to chronic hypoxia in the brain and heart tissues, in absence of Epo. The first part will briefly describe the similarities of the signaling process of hypoxia-induced angiogenesis, as well as the other mechanisms that take place to protect the brain and heart against anemic and hypoxic injuries. The second part will focus on these adaptations in response to chronic anemia due to Epo deficiency (in comparison with adaptations induced by hypoxia). The third part will mainly describe the effect of both constraints (anemia and hypoxia) in cerebral and cardiac tissues.

2. Adaptations to chronic hypoxia in cerebral and cardiac tissues

2.1. Brain under chronic hypoxia

In the central nervous system, cerebrovascular and energy metabolism adaptations occur under hypoxic conditions in order to preserve an adequate tissue oxygen supply needed to support an optimal neuronal function. An acute hypoxic exposure triggers both a CBF and glucose consumption increases [18]. The stabilization of HIF-1α rapidly up regulates the vaso-dilatory enzyme inducible nitric oxide synthase (iNOS) [19]. NO, the enzymatic product of iNOS, relaxes vascular smooth muscle cells, providing a short-term increase in blood flow. Thus, an increase in cerebral NO following a rise in NOS isoforms expression is most probably responsible for the rise in CBF [20–23]. With longer hypoxic exposure, polycythemia and cerebral angiogenesis take place to enhance cerebral oxygenation, while cerebral NO level returns to basal value [23, 24]. Indeed, in a chronic hypoxic challenge to the central nervous system, the cerebral cortex is known to undergo a significant cerebrovascular remodeling, in order to preserve tissue oxygen and energy supply [24–29]. These microvascular changes occur relatively late compared to the physiological adaptations [30]. In the rat brain, the capillary density almost doubles, and the average intercapillary distance decreases from about 50 to about 40 μm [31]. Also, by 3 weeks of adaptation, the initial hypoxic-induced increased flow returns to baseline by 5 days [22], concomitantly there is an increasing hematocrit, glucose consumption is slightly elevated by about 15% [32–34] and tissue oxygen tension is restored [35, 36]. Finally, it is well accepted that blood flow alterations serve acute changes in oxygen delivery, while persistent changes are due to capillary density adjustments.

Molecular mechanisms underlying hypoxia-induced capillary increases are now well documented and involve specifically HIF-1α/VEGF pathway [23, 26, 33, 37, 38]. The HIF pathway regulates a host of pro-angiogenic genes, including VEGF, angiopoietin-1, angiopoietin-2 (Ang-2) and many others [39, 40]. HIF-regulated pro-angiogenic factors execute the HIF-specific angiogenic program by increasing vascular permeability (most probably through interaction with NO [41]), endothelial cell proliferation, sprouting, migration, adhesion and tube formation. In rats, HIF-1α is detected in the brain, in all cell types, shortly after the onset of hypoxia and persists for at least 2 weeks, until cerebral angiogenesis is completed within 3 weeks of exposure to hypoxia [23, 29, 35]. Brain angiogenesis also requires additional pro-angiogenic factors such as Ang-2. Ang-2, which is not constitutively expressed under normoxic conditions, is upregulated in rat and mouse endothelial cells following hypoxia [28, 38]. Ang-2 induction during hypoxia is known to occur independently of HIF-1 and is due to cyclooxygenase-2 (COX-2) enzyme activity [42, 43]. More recent results also demonstrated that the hypoxic capillary response in aged mice was preserved after 3 weeks of hypoxia despite a significant delay in the response during the first week of exposure to hypoxia [25].

2.2. Heart under chronic hypoxia

In humans, the most characteristic and important cardiovascular response to hypoxia is pulmonary vasoconstriction, which reduces the caliber of pulmonary vessels and raises vascular resistance in a region of low alveolar PO_2. However, severe hypoxia has a direct deleterious effect on cardiac function. Hypoxic pulmonary vasoconstriction can cause chronic pulmonary hypertension. Myocardial contractility and maximum output are diminished during conditions of reduced oxygen supply. While maximum oxygen consumption is reduced in chronic hypoxia, cardiac output (CO) remains normal at rest, owing primarily to an increased red blood cell mass [44, 45].

In our animal model, we showed that all parameters of cardiac function were preserved when comparing wild-type (WT) mice under normoxic and chronic hypoxic conditions. Indeed, systolic blood pressure was not affected by 14-day hypoxia at 4500 m, and hypoxic wild-type mice did not develop pulmonary hypertension. Moreover, there was no cardiac hypertrophy at variance with what was shown in rats or humans in similar hypoxic conditions [46]. Moreover, cardiac output was not affected by chronic hypoxia alone and oxygen delivery was maintained. In addition, hypoxic wild-type mice responded by increasing plasma Epo and blood hemoglobin, resulting in a rise in oxygen-carrying capacity [47].

Furthermore, many reports now stated that heart could be an additional Epo productive tissue [48, 49]. Hoch et al. first showed an Epo gene and protein expression in cardiac progenitor cells [50]. Through specific binding to its receptor EpoR, Epo triggers intracellular signaling events that depend on the activation of Jak2 tyrosine kinase [51]. The exploration of these pathways revealed that Epo is also an angiogenic as well as an anti-apoptotic factor as described respectively in the brain [52] and the heart [47, 50, 53, 54]. As previously described [55], chronic hypoxia led to the activation of HIF-1α/VEGF pathway in the heart of adult wild-type mice most probably responsible for their enhanced myocardial angiogenesis. Also we demonstrated the activation of cardioprotective pathways, involving HIF-1α and Epo, as suggested by the increase of EpoR expression and P-STAT-5/STAT-5 ratio [47]. Furthermore, we could not exclude a cardiac metabolic gene remodeling since temporal changes in glucose metabolic genes in response to moderate hypobaric hypoxia [56] have been demonstrated.

However, these adaptive responses contribute to maintain an adequate tissue oxygen supply for the preservation of cardiac function and to protect the heart against hypoxic insults.

3. Adaptations to chronic Epo deficiency in cerebral and cardiac tissues

Anemia is defined as a lack of oxygen-carrying red blood cells which also results in a lack of oxygen delivery to tissue. The physiological and molecular responses to tissue hypoxia are increasingly understood while the effects of anemia are still poorly documented [57]. Our model of erythropoietin-SV40 T antigen (Epo-TAg[h]) transgenic mice presents a severe reduction of Epo expression that induces chronic anemia [16, 17]. The first studies demonstrated that Epo-Tag[h] mice could survive in chronic hypoxia (14 days at 4500 m), in part through an increase in ventilation and probably a higher cardiac output as suggested by a significant cardiac hypertrophy [58–60]. Hence, it was of interest of our team to compare the physiological and cellular responses to chronic anemia (low Hb) and chronic hypoxia (low P_aO_2) in cerebral and cardiac tissues. Indeed, the objectives of our studies were to determine if chronic anemic mice developed compensatory mechanisms in the brain and heart (vascular remodeling, adaptative function, pathways involving HIF-1α) to offset the decrease in hemoglobin concentration.

3.1. Brain under chronic anemia

Low O_2 environment is the principal regulator of HIF activity. The HIF pathway mediates the primary cellular responses to low O_2, which promotes both short- and long-term adaptation to hypoxia as already described in the previous paragraph. In this regard, we considered that anemia-induced cerebral hypoxia involved the same hypoxic molecules. It has already been described that anemia increases cerebral hypoxic genes expression such as HIF, VEGF and nNOS which are involved in O_2 homeostasis [61]. Indeed, studies on severe hemodilution using NOS-deficient mice showed an increased expression of HIF and nNOS proteins in the brain as well as an increased whole body HIF activity [57, 61–64]. Many other molecules, including Epo, VEGF and iNOS have also been shown to be upregulated in the anemic brain [61, 65]. Thus, it seems that during anemia, HIF-1α has the potential to regulate cerebral cellular responses under both hypoxic and normoxic conditions [23, 47, 57, 64, 65].

Then, we focused on potential mediators of the increase in CBF associated with both hypoxia and anemia. Indeed, local production of NO by endothelial NOS (eNOS), and nNOS mediates CBF under a number of physiological conditions, including anemia and hypoxia [24, 61, 63, 64]. Relatively specific inhibition of nNOS has been demonstrated to impair the increase in CBF associated with acute anemia [61] and hypoxia [66–68], implicating nNOS as an important mediator of CBF in both cases [63, 64]. In our studies, we also found an increase in nNOS, while iNOS and eNOS were unchanged but no corresponding change in cerebral NO concentration. The stabilization of HIF-1α, as already described in the brain in acute [61, 69] and chronic anemia [23], promote VEGF-induced angiogenesis as shown in normoxic Epo-TAg[h] mice with a rise in the capillary/fiber ratio, thus optimizing oxygen diffusion as previously described in the brain [24]. Erythropoietin also plays an important role in angiogenesis through upregulation of VEGF in ischemic rats [11]. Indeed, Wang et al. showed that neural progenitor cells treated with Epo were able to produce VEGF and consequently to promote angiogenesis through the upregulation of VEGFR2 expression in cerebral endothelial cells [70].

Our work provided novel physiological data about cerebral adaptations to chronic anemia. Indeed, we evidenced that Epo deficiency activated cerebral hypoxic mechanisms through HIF activation that promote angiogenesis [23]. In addition, the JAK/STAT signaling pathway mediated by the Epo/EpoR complex seems to be activated by chronic anemia [23, 47] and could promote neuroprotection and cell proliferation [71]. Furthermore, more recent results showed that nNOS is specifically protective during anemia [57]. All these responses were probably able to minimize brain damage that could be induced by chronic anemia. Finally, the mechanisms responsible for matching capillary density to tissue oxygen levels are not unique to environmental hypoxic stimuli. Rather, these processes appear to be responsible for maintaining the oxygen availability through local blood flow in order to optimize the neuronal function.

3.2. Heart under chronic anemia

The classic physiological cardiovascular responses to anemia include an increased CO, a redistribution of blood flow and a decrease of hemoglobin-oxygen affinity. Two mechanisms are most probably responsible for the increased CO during anemia: reduced blood viscosity and increased sympathetic stimulation of the cardiovascular effectors. Blood viscosity affects both preload and afterload, two of the major determinants of the CO, whereas sympathetic stimulation primarily increases heart rate and contractility [72]. If cardiac function is normal, the increase in venous return or left ventricular preload will be the most important determinant of the increased CO during normovolemic anemia [72]. It is also known that anemia induces right and left ventricular hypertrophy [59, 73, 74] and increases CO, offsetting the fall in arterial oxygen content to maintain oxygen delivery. Our data confirmed the increase in CO by an increase in the stroke volume associated with a left ventricular dilatation as expected by Olivetti et al. [74]. Taken together, these data suggest that the enhancement in CO could be explained by both an increase in preload and autonomous nervous system stimulation. Indeed, our data showed an increase in myocardial function parameters in normoxic anemic mice. However, although the CO was increased in Epo-Tag^h mice, oxygen delivery remained lower than in controls. This could induce the stabilization of the transcription factor HIF-1α as already described in the brain in both models of acute and chronic anemia [61, 69]. This stabilization promotes VEGF-induced angiogenesis as shown in normoxic Epo-TAg^h mice with a rise in the capillaries/fibers ratio, thus optimizing oxygen diffusion as described in the brain [24]. This increase in capillary density could allow the development of cardiac hypertrophy without myocardial dysfunction, as previously described in rats in a model of anemia induced by iron-deficient diet [74]. Furthermore, we could not exclude that increased expression of nNOS also contributed to these adaptive cardiovascular responses in chronic anemic mice. Indeed, acute anemia resulted in an increase in CO and a reduced stroke volume in WT anemic mice while in contrast, CO and stroke volume responses were severely attenuated in anemic nNOS$^{-/-}$ mice [57]. In addition, a model of *Hif1a*$^{+/-}$ hemizigous mice revealed impaired increases in hematocrit, right ventricular mass and right ventricular pressure, allowing us to speculate that increased HIF-1α may have participated in these physiological responses to anemia in our model [75].

4. Effects of chronic anemia and hypoxia on cerebral and cardiac tissues

As previously explained, plethora of studies are available to describe cerebral and cardiac adaptations and their underlying molecular mechanisms in response to chronic hypoxia or anemia separately. Our group investigated for the first time, the effects of chronic hypobaric hypoxia combined with chronic anemia in the heart and brain of the transgenic Epo-TAg[h] mice. So far, the few studies from other groups that also use transgenic mice overexpressing Epo (Tg6 and Tg21) display results that are complementary to our data but also more detailed. Indeed, these studies also describe the pathways involved in the ventilatory responses to hypoxia and aim to clarify the role of Epo in respiratory acclimatization to hypoxia at physiological, cellular and molecular levels. Even though, we were not able to find other animal studies combining the effects of both chronic hypoxia and anemia on cardiac or cerebral tissues, comparing studies at a multidisciplinary level may provide new approaches and therapies for diseases associated with hypoxia.

4.1. Brain under chronic hypoxia and anemia

In the brain, both Epo and its receptor are upregulated during ischaemia/hypoxia [76, 77] and Epo administration considerably inhibits apoptosis after middle cerebral artery occlusion [78]. Apart from its positive effects in acute ischaemic brain damage, Epo is a potent stimulator of the hypoxic ventilatory response (HVR) by interacting with respiratory centers in the brainstem [79]. Indeed, the blockade of Epo's activity in the brainstem of adult C57Bl6 mice by intracisternal injections of the soluble Epo receptor (sEpoR) induced a reduction of the basal minute ventilation, but it did not affect the central chemosensitivity [80, 81]. In contrast, recent study using transgenic mice Tg6 (that present a human Epo gene overexpression in brain and circulation; Tg21: Epo overexpression in brain) suggested that Epo blunts the HVR through an interaction with central and peripheral respiratory chemocenters [81]. In our model, acute hypoxic ventilatory response was increased after chronic hypoxia in wild-type mice but remained unchanged in Epo-TAg[h] mice, confirming that adequate erythropoietin level is necessary to obtain an appropriate HVR and a significant ventilatory acclimatization to hypoxia. Surprisingly, both constraints (chronic hypoxia and anemia) did not trigger a synergic effect in any studied parameters except a high cerebral NO level that could suggest an improved brain perfusion. Finally, the response to chronic hypoxia was divergent in the brain of wild-type and anemic mice. Indeed, these adaptation processes including angiogenesis and neuroprotection were globally altered in Epo-TAg[h] mice exposed to chronic hypoxia.

Taken together, all these data suggest that Epo/EpoR pathways activation is necessary to initiate neuroprotection mechanisms as well as cerebral angiogenesis under hypoxia but also might help to better understand respiratory disorders at high altitude.

4.2. Heart under chronic hypoxia and anemia

Independently, chronic anemia and chronic hypoxia increased the expression of HIF-1α, VEGF and Epo, cytokines that are involved in both angiogenesis and cardioprotection through specific signaling pathways acting to compensate oxygen transport deficiency. Recent studies also involved these same cytokines in the cardiovascular responses as well as increased cardiac output observed in acute anemia [57, 75]. Our data showed a decrease in left ventricular hypertrophy and functional left ventricular adaptation as well as a reduced oxygen delivery in the heart of hypoxic Epo-TAg[h] mice. Results from other groups showed that Tg6 mice did not develop pulmonary hypertension in normoxia or after exposure to chronic hypoxia (10% O_2 for 3 weeks) [82] suggesting an important role of Epo in functional adaptation of the heart to chronic hypoxia. Similarly to what occurred in the brain, we did not observe a synergic effect of these combined constraints on the expression of the hypoxic genes in the heart of chronically hypoxic Epo-TAg[h] mice suggesting that adaptive responses to both constraints are already maximal. However, the increased P-STAT-5/STAT-5 ratio is concordant with a direct protective effect of Epo on cardiomyocytes and endothelial cells as well as stimulation of angiogenesis in the ischaemic heart [83]. Capillary density was unchanged in spite of the fall in HIF-1α/VEGF pathway probably because the initiation of the capillarization with acute hypoxia necessitates VEGF, while its maintenance in chronic hypoxia involves other factors such as angiopoietins [38, 43].

Taken together, our results suggest that adaptative mechanisms that take place with chronic anemia are somewhat similar to those in response to 14 days of hypoxia. However, when both constraints are applied, these mechanisms failed to maintain an adequate cardiac adaptation with a secondary decrease in body oxygen supply, despite the activation of cardioprotective pathways.

5. Perspectives and significance

In this review, a proposal is made that chronic anemia-induced hypoxia triggers regulatory pathways that mediate long-term adaptive cardiac and cerebral changes, particularly at the transcriptional level. These adaptative mechanisms include a regulated increase in cerebral blood flow, cardiac output, angiogenesis and cytoprotection triggered by HIF-1α, VEGF and Epo pathways. All these compensatory mechanisms aim to optimize oxygen delivery and to protect the brain and heart from hypoxic injury to allow acclimatization. However, when both arterial pressure and content of oxygen are decreased, the cerebral and cardiac adaptative mechanisms showed their limitations. We could not exclude that cerebral and cardiac cell injuries occurred following the combined effect of chronic anemia and hypoxia as well as of the NO toxicity. **Figure 1** summarizes the cerebral and cardiac plasticity induced by chronic anemia and/or hypoxia. Data shown in this figure are all based on animal studies. Moreover, a recent review of our group includes also ventilatory [60], muscular [84, 85] and rheologic [86] adaptations in this model of mice. Finally, investigating the molecular mechanisms of O_2 homeostasis represents a mean of gaining new insights to the hypoxia-induced cerebral and myocardial injuries. But it is of great clinical importance to study extensively these non-erythropoietic functions of Epo to contribute to the development of new therapeutic strategies for the management of brain and heart ischemia.

Figure 1 summarizes the physiological adaptations to chronic hypoxia and anemia in the heart and brain of our model of Epo-TAg[h] mice. The green color represents the responses of normoxic anemic mice. The blue color represents the responses of hypoxic control mice. The red color represents the responses of hypoxic anemic mice. The arrows represent an increase or decrease of the response, while the '=' symbol means no change between normoxia and hypoxia. PaO_2 is arterial pressure of oxygen, CaO_2 is arterial content of oxygen, PiO_2 is inspired pressure of oxygen and TO_2 is transport of oxygen.

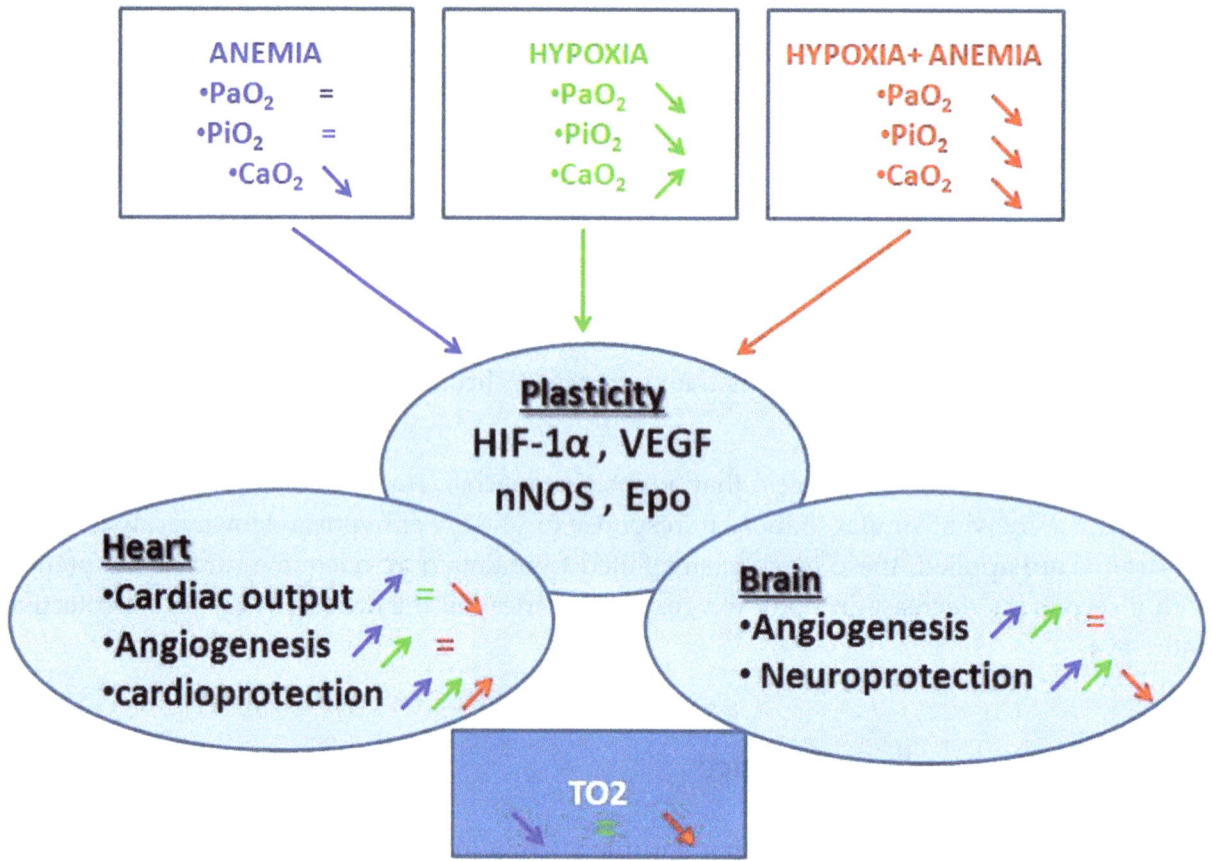

Figure 1. Cerebral and cardiac plasticity induced by chronic anemia and/or hypoxia in Epo-Tag^h mice.

Grants

All the original articles of our group cited in this review were supported by "Agence Nationale de la Recherche" n°ANR-08-GENOPAT-029.

Author details

Raja El Hasnaoui-Saadani

Address all correspondence to: rajaelhasnaoui@hotmail.com

Research center-College of Medicine- Princess Nourah bint Abdulrahmane University, Riyadh, Saudi Arabia

References

[1] Semenza GL. Vascular responses to hypoxia and ischemia. Arteriosclerosis, thrombosis, and vascular biology. 2010 Apr;30(4):648–52. PubMed PMID: 19729615. Pubmed Central PMCID: 2841694.

[2] Ehrenreich H, Hasselblatt M, Dembowski C, Cepek L, Lewczuk P, Stiefel M, et al. Erythropoietin therapy for acute stroke is both safe and beneficial. Molecular medicine. 2002 Aug;8(8):495–505. PubMed PMID: 12435860. Pubmed Central PMCID: 2040012.

[3] Ehrenreich H, Weissenborn K, Prange H, Schneider D, Weimar C, Wartenberg K, et al. Recombinant human erythropoietin in the treatment of acute ischemic stroke. Stroke; a journal of cerebral circulation. 2009 Dec;40(12):e647–56. PubMed PMID: 19834012.

[4] Cohen R, Shainberg A, Hochhauser E, Cheporko Y, Tobar A, Birk E, et al. UTP reduces infarct size and improves mice heart function after myocardial infarct via P2Y2 receptor. Biochemical pharmacology. 2011 Nov 1;82(9):1126–33. PubMed PMID: 21839729.

[5] Forsythe JA, Jiang BH, Iyer NV, Agani F, Leung SW, Koos RD, et al. Activation of vascular endothelial growth factor gene transcription by hypoxia-inducible factor 1. Molecular and cellular biology. 1996 Sep;16(9):4604-13. PubMed PMID: 8756616. Pubmed Central PMCID: 231459.

[6] Gassmann M, Heinicke K, Soliz J, Ogunshola OO. Non-erythroid functions of erythropoietin. Advances in experimental medicine and biology. 2003;543:323–30. PubMed PMID: 14713131.

[7] Vogel J, Gassmann M. Erythropoietic and non-erythropoietic functions of erythropoietin in mouse models. The journal of physiology. 2011 Mar 15;589(Pt 6):1259–64. PubMed PMID: 21282290. Pubmed Central PMCID: 3082089.

[8] Wu H, Lee SH, Gao J, Liu X, Iruela-Arispe ML. Inactivation of erythropoietin leads to defects in cardiac morphogenesis. Development. 1999 Aug;126(16):3597–605. PubMed PMID: 10409505.

[9] Liu C, Shen K, Liu Z, Noguchi CT. Regulated human erythropoietin receptor expression in mouse brain. The journal of biological chemistry. 1997 Dec 19;272(51):32395–400. PubMed PMID: 9405448.

[10] Chen ZY, Warin R, Noguchi CT. Erythropoietin and normal brain development: receptor expression determines multi-tissue response. Neuro-degenerative diseases. 2006;3(1–2):68–75. PubMed PMID: 16909040.

[11] Wang L, Zhang Z, Wang Y, Zhang R, Chopp M. Treatment of stroke with erythropoietin enhances neurogenesis and angiogenesis and improves neurological function in rats. Stroke; a journal of cerebral circulation. 2004 Jul;35(7):1732–7. PubMed PMID: 15178821.

[12] Ribatti D, Vacca A, Roccaro AM, Crivellato E, Presta M. Erythropoietin as an angiogenic factor. European journal of clinical investigation. 2003 Oct;33(10):891–6. PubMed PMID: 14511361.

[13] Marti HH, Bernaudin M, Petit E, Bauer C. Neuroprotection and angiogenesis: dual role of erythropoietin in brain ischemia. News in physiological sciences: an international journal

of physiology produced jointly by the International Union of Physiological Sciences and the American Physiological Society. 2000 Oct;15:225–9. PubMed PMID: 11390915.

[14] Jaquet K, Krause K, Tawakol-Khodai M, Geidel S, Kuck KH. Erythropoietin and VEGF exhibit equal angiogenic potential. Microvascular research. 2002 Sep;64(2):326–33. PubMed PMID: 12204656.

[15] Xiong Y, Mahmood A, Meng Y, Zhang Y, Qu C, Schallert T, et al. Delayed administration of erythropoietin reducing hippocampal cell loss, enhancing angiogenesis and neurogenesis, and improving functional outcome following traumatic brain injury in rats: comparison of treatment with single and triple dose. Journal of neurosurgery. 2010 Sep;113(3):598–608. PubMed PMID: 19817538. Pubmed Central PMCID: 2898921.

[16] Maxwell PH, Osmond MK, Pugh CW, Heryet A, Nicholls LG, Tan CC, et al. Identification of the renal erythropoietin-producing cells using transgenic mice. Kidney international. 1993 Nov;44(5):1149–62. PubMed PMID: 8264149.

[17] Binley K, Askham Z, Iqball S, Spearman H, Martin L, de Alwis M, et al. Long-term reversal of chronic anemia using a hypoxia-regulated erythropoietin gene therapy. Blood. 2002 Oct 1;100(7):2406–13. PubMed PMID: 12239150.

[18] Xu K, Lamanna JC. Chronic hypoxia and the cerebral circulation. Journal of applied physiology. 2006 Feb;100(2):725–30. PubMed PMID: 16421279.

[19] Yin JH, Yang DI, Ku G, Hsu CY. iNOS expression inhibits hypoxia-inducible factor-1 activity. Biochemical and biophysical research communications. 2000 Dec 9;279(1):30–4. PubMed PMID: 11112413.

[20] Hudetz AG, Shen H, Kampine JP. Nitric oxide from neuronal NOS plays critical role in cerebral capillary flow response to hypoxia. The American journal of physiology. 1998 Mar;274(3 Pt 2):H982-9. PubMed PMID: 9530212.

[21] LaManna JC, McCracken KA, Strohl KP. Changes in regional cerebral blood flow and sucrose space after 3-4 weeks of hypobaric hypoxia (0.5 ATM). Advances in experimental medicine and biology. 1989;248:471–7. PubMed PMID: 2506740.

[22] LaManna JC. Rat brain adaptation to chronic hypobaric hypoxia. Advances in experimental medicine and biology. 1992;317:107–14. PubMed PMID: 1288116.

[23] El Hasnaoui-Saadani R, Pichon A, Marchant D, Olivier P, Launay T, Quidu P, et al. Cerebral adaptations to chronic anemia in a model of erythropoietin-deficient mice exposed to hypoxia. American journal of physiology regulatory, integrative and comparative physiology. 2009 Mar;296(3):R801–11. PubMed PMID: 19109375.

[24] LaManna JC, Chavez JC, Pichiule P. Structural and functional adaptation to hypoxia in the rat brain. The Journal of experimental biology. 2004 Aug;207(Pt 18):3163–9. PubMed PMID: 15299038.

[25] Benderro GF, Sun X, Kuang Y, Lamanna JC. Decreased VEGF expression and micro-vascular density, but increased HIF-1 and 2alpha accumulation and EPO expression in chronic moderate hyperoxia in the mouse brain. Brain research. 2012 Aug 30;1471:46–55. PubMed PMID: 22820296. Pubmed Central PMCID: 3454487.

[26] Boero JA, Ascher J, Arregui A, Rovainen C, Woolsey TA. Increased brain capillaries in chronic hypoxia. Journal of applied physiology. 1999 Apr;86(4):1211–9. PubMed PMID: 10194205.

[27] Dore-Duffy P, LaManna JC. Physiologic angiodynamics in the brain. Antioxidants & redox signaling. 2007 Sep;9(9):1363–71. PubMed PMID: 17627476.

[28] Ward NL, Moore E, Noon K, Spassil N, Keenan E, Ivanco TL, et al. Cerebral angiogenic factors, angiogenesis, and physiological response to chronic hypoxia differ among four commonly used mouse strains. Journal of applied physiology. 2007 May;102(5):1927–35. PubMed PMID: 17234796.

[29] Pichiule P, Agani F, Chavez JC, Xu K, LaManna JC. HIF-1 alpha and VEGF expression after transient global cerebral ischemia. Advances in experimental medicine and biology. 2003;530:611–7. PubMed PMID: 14562758.

[30] Xu K, Puchowicz MA, LaManna JC. Renormalization of regional brain blood flow during prolonged mild hypoxic exposure in rats. Brain research. 2004 Nov 19;1027(1-2):188–91. PubMed PMID: 15494170.

[31] Lauro KL, LaManna JC. Adequacy of cerebral vascular remodeling following three weeks of hypobaric hypoxia. Examined by an integrated composite analytical model. Advances in experimental medicine and biology. 1997;411:369–76. PubMed PMID: 9269451.

[32] Pelligrino DA, LaManna JC, Duckrow RB, Bryan RM, Jr., Harik SI. Hyperglycemia and blood-brain barrier glucose transport. Journal of cerebral blood flow and metabolism: official journal of the International Society of Cerebral Blood Flow and Metabolism. 1992 Nov;12(6):887–99. PubMed PMID: 1400643.

[33] Harik SI, Hritz MA, LaManna JC. Hypoxia-induced brain angiogenesis in the adult rat. The journal of physiology. 1995 Jun 1;485 (Pt 2):525–30. PubMed PMID: 7545234. Pubmed Central PMCID: 1158011.

[34] Harik SI, Lust WD, Jones SC, Lauro KL, Pundik S, LaManna JC. Brain glucose metabolism in hypobaric hypoxia. Journal of applied physiology. 1995 Jul;79(1):136–40. PubMed PMID: 7559210.

[35] Chavez JC, Agani F, Pichiule P, LaManna JC. Expression of hypoxia-inducible factor-1alpha in the brain of rats during chronic hypoxia. Journal of applied physiology. 2000 Nov;89(5):1937–42. PubMed PMID: 11053346.

[36] Dunn JF, Grinberg O, Roche M, Nwaigwe CI, Hou HG, Swartz HM. Noninvasive assessment of cerebral oxygenation during acclimation to hypobaric hypoxia. Journal of cerebral

blood flow and metabolism: official journal of the International Society of Cerebral Blood Flow and Metabolism. 2000 Dec;20(12):1632–5. PubMed PMID: 11129779.

[37] Mironov V, Hritz MA, LaManna JC, Hudetz AG, Harik SI. Architectural alterations in rat cerebral microvessels after hypobaric hypoxia. Brain research. 1994 Oct 10;660(1):73–80. PubMed PMID: 7828003.

[38] Pichiule P, LaManna JC. Angiopoietin-2 and rat brain capillary remodeling during adaptation and deadaptation to prolonged mild hypoxia. Journal of applied physiology. 2002 Sep;93(3):1131–9. PubMed PMID: 12183511.

[39] Krock BL, Skuli N, Simon MC. Hypoxia-induced angiogenesis: good and evil. Genes & cancer. 2011 Dec;2(12):1117–33. PubMed PMID: 22866203. Pubmed Central PMCID: 3411127.

[40] Fong GH. Mechanisms of adaptive angiogenesis to tissue hypoxia. Angiogenesis. 2008;11(2):121–40. PubMed PMID: 18327686.

[41] Agani FH, Puchowicz M, Chavez JC, Pichiule P, LaManna J. Role of nitric oxide in the regulation of HIF-1alpha expression during hypoxia. American journal of physiology cell physiology. 2002 Jul;283(1):C178–86. PubMed PMID: 12055086.

[42] Kanaan A, Farahani R, Douglas RM, Lamanna JC, Haddad GG. Effect of chronic continuous or intermittent hypoxia and reoxygenation on cerebral capillary density and myelination. American journal of physiology regulatory, integrative and comparative physiology. 2006 Apr;290(4):R1105–14. PubMed PMID: 16322350.

[43] Pichiule P, Chavez JC, LaManna JC. Hypoxic regulation of angiopoietin-2 expression in endothelial cells. The journal of biological chemistry. 2004 Mar 26;279(13):12171–80. PubMed PMID: 14702352.

[44] Banchero N. Cardiovascular responses to chronic hypoxia. Annual review of physiology. 1987;49:465–76. PubMed PMID: 3551810.

[45] Pierson DJ. Pathophysiology and clinical effects of chronic hypoxia. Respiratory care. 2000 Jan;45(1):39–51; discussion-3. PubMed PMID: 10771781.

[46] Leon-Velarde F, Villafuerte FC, Richalet JP. Chronic mountain sickness and the heart. Progress in cardiovascular diseases. 2010 May–Jun;52(6):540–9. PubMed PMID: 20417348.

[47] El Hasnaoui-Saadani R, Marchant D, Pichon A, Escoubet B, Pezet M, Hilfiker-Kleiner D, et al. Epo deficiency alters cardiac adaptation to chronic hypoxia. Respiratory physiology & neurobiology. 2013 Apr 1;186(2):146–54. PubMed PMID: 23333855.

[48] Bin-Jaliah I, Ammar HI, Mikhailidis DP, Dallak MA, Al-Hashem FH, Haidara MA, et al. Cardiac adaptive responses after hypoxia in an experimental model. Angiology. 2010 Feb;61(2):145–56. PubMed PMID: 19939823.

[49] Cai Z, Semenza GL. Phosphatidylinositol-3-kinase signaling is required for erythropoietin-mediated acute protection against myocardial ischemia/reperfusion injury. Circulation. 2004 May 4;109(17):2050–3. PubMed PMID: 15117842.

[50] Hoch M, Fischer P, Stapel B, Missol-Kolka E, Sekkali B, Scherr M, et al. Erythropoietin preserves the endothelial differentiation capacity of cardiac progenitor cells and reduces heart failure during anticancer therapies. Cell stem cell. 2011 Aug 5;9(2):131–43. PubMed PMID: 21816364.

[51] Koury MJ, Bondurant MC. The molecular mechanism of erythropoietin action. European journal of biochemistry/FEBS. 1992 Dec 15;210(3):649–63. PubMed PMID: 1483451.

[52] Digicaylioglu M, Lipton SA. Erythropoietin-mediated neuroprotection involves cross-talk between Jak2 and NF-kappaB signalling cascades. Nature. 2001 Aug 9;412(6847):641–7. PubMed PMID: 11493922.

[53] Kertesz N, Wu J, Chen TH, Sucov HM, Wu H. The role of erythropoietin in regulating angiogenesis. Developmental biology. 2004 Dec 1;276(1):101–10. PubMed PMID: 15531367.

[54] Marzo F, Lavorgna A, Coluzzi G, Santucci E, Tarantino F, Rio T, et al. Erythropoietin in heart and vessels: focus on transcription and signalling pathways. Journal of thrombosis and thrombolysis. 2008 Dec;26(3):183–7. PubMed PMID: 18338108.

[55] Ray PS, Estrada-Hernandez T, Sasaki H, Zhu L, Maulik N. Early effects of hypoxia/reoxygenation on VEGF, ang-1, ang-2 and their receptors in the rat myocardium: implications for myocardial angiogenesis. Molecular and cellular biochemistry. 2000 Oct;213(1–2):145–53. PubMed PMID: 11129953.

[56] Sharma S, Taegtmeyer H, Adrogue J, Razeghi P, Sen S, Ngumbela K, et al. Dynamic changes of gene expression in hypoxia-induced right ventricular hypertrophy. American journal of physiology heart and circulatory physiology. 2004 Mar;286(3):H1185–92. PubMed PMID: 14630626.

[57] Tsui AK, Marsden PA, Mazer CD, Adamson SL, Henkelman RM, Ho JJ, et al. Priming of hypoxia-inducible factor by neuronal nitric oxide synthase is essential for adaptive responses to severe anemia. Proceedings of the National Academy of Sciences of the United States of America. 2011 Oct 18;108(42):17544–9. PubMed PMID: 21976486. Pubmed Central PMCID: 3198321.

[58] Macarlupu JL, Buvry A, Morel OE, Leon-Velarde F, Richalet JP, Favret F. Time course of ventilatory acclimatisation to hypoxia in a model of anemic transgenic mice. Respiratory physiology & neurobiology. 2006 Aug;153(1):14–22. PubMed PMID: 16330260.

[59] Macarlupu JL, Buvry A, Morel OE, Leon-Velarde F, Richalet JP, Favret F. Characterisation of the ventilatory response to hypoxia in a model of transgenic anemic mice. Respiratory physiology & neurobiology. 2006 Jan 25;150(1):19–26. PubMed PMID: 15878311.

[60] Voituron N, Jeton F, Cholley Y, Hasnaoui-Saadani RE, Marchant D, Quidu P, et al. Catalyzing role of erythropoietin on the nitric oxide central pathway during the ventilatory responses to hypoxia. Physiological reports. 2014 Feb 1;2(2):e00223. PubMed PMID: 24744892. Pubmed Central PMCID: 3966246.

[61] McLaren AT, Marsden PA, Mazer CD, Baker AJ, Stewart DJ, Tsui AK, et al. Increased expression of HIF-1alpha, nNOS, and VEGF in the cerebral cortex of anemic rats. American journal of physiology Regulatory, integrative and comparative physiology. 2007 Jan;292(1):R403–14. PubMed PMID: 16973934.

[62] Hare GM, Mazer CD, Hutchison JS, McLaren AT, Liu E, Rassouli A, et al. Severe hemodilutional anemia increases cerebral tissue injury following acute neurotrauma. Journal of applied physiology. 2007 Sep;103(3):1021–9. PubMed PMID: 17556499.

[63] Hare GM, Mazer CD, Mak W, Gorczynski RM, Hum KM, Kim SY, et al. Hemodilutional anemia is associated with increased cerebral neuronal nitric oxide synthase gene expression. Journal of applied physiology. 2003 May;94(5):2058–67. PubMed PMID: 12533500.

[64] Hare GM, Tsui AK, McLaren AT, Ragoonanan TE, Yu J, Mazer CD. Anemia and cerebral outcomes: many questions, fewer answers. Anesthesia and analgesia. 2008 Oct;107(4):1356–70. PubMed PMID: 18806052.

[65] Tsui AK, Marsden PA, Mazer CD, Sled JG, Lee KM, Henkelman RM, et al. Differential HIF and NOS responses to acute anemia: defining organ-specific hemoglobin thresholds for tissue hypoxia. American journal of physiology Regulatory, integrative and comparative physiology. 2014 Jul 1;307(1):R13–25. PubMed PMID: 24760996.

[66] Pearce WJ. Mechanisms of hypoxic cerebral vasodilatation. Pharmacology & therapeutics. 1995 Jan;65(1):75–91. PubMed PMID: 7716183.

[67] Serrano J, Encinas JM, Salas E, Fernandez AP, Castro-Blanco S, Fernandez-Vizarra P, et al. Hypobaric hypoxia modifies constitutive nitric oxide synthase activity and protein nitration in the rat cerebellum. Brain research. 2003 Jun 20;976(1):109–19. PubMed PMID: 12763628.

[68] Serrano J, Encinas JM, Fernandez AP, Rodrigo J, Martinez A. Effects of acute hypobaric hypoxia on the nitric oxide system of the rat cerebral cortex: Protective role of nitric oxide inhibitors. Neuroscience. 2006 Oct 27;142(3):799–808. PubMed PMID: 16952423.

[69] Rakusan K, Cicutti N, Kolar F. Effect of anemia on cardiac function, microvascular structure, and capillary hematocrit in rat hearts. American journal of physiology Heart and circulatory physiology. 2001 Mar;280(3):H1407–14. PubMed PMID: 11179091.

[70] Wang L, Chopp M, Gregg SR, Zhang RL, Teng H, Jiang A, et al. Neural progenitor cells treated with EPO induce angiogenesis through the production of VEGF. Journal of cerebral blood flow and metabolism: official journal of the International Society of Cerebral Blood Flow and Metabolism. 2008 Jul;28(7):1361–8. PubMed PMID: 18414495. Pubmed Central PMCID: 3971950.

[71] Lopez TV, Lappin TR, Maxwell P, Shi Z, Lopez-Marure R, Aguilar C, et al. Autocrine/paracrine erythropoietin signalling promotes JAK/STAT-dependent proliferation of human cervical cancer cells. International journal of cancer. 2011 Dec 1;129(11):2566–76. PubMed PMID: 21442620.

[72] Hebert PC, Van der Linden P, Biro G, Hu LQ. Physiologic aspects of anemia. Critical care clinics. 2004 Apr;20(2):187–212. PubMed PMID: 15135460.

[73] Naito Y, Tsujino T, Matsumoto M, Sakoda T, Ohyanagi M, Masuyama T. Adaptive response of the heart to long-term anemia induced by iron deficiency. American journal of physiology heart and circulatory physiology. 2009 Mar;296(3):H585–93. PubMed PMID: 19136608.

[74] Olivetti G, Lagrasta C, Quaini F, Ricci R, Moccia G, Capasso JM, et al. Capillary growth in anemia-induced ventricular wall remodeling in the rat heart. Circulation research. 1989 Nov;65(5):1182–92. PubMed PMID: 2529998.

[75] Yu AY, Shimoda LA, Iyer NV, Huso DL, Sun X, McWilliams R, et al. Impaired physiological responses to chronic hypoxia in mice partially deficient for hypoxia-inducible factor 1alpha. The journal of clinical investigation. 1999 Mar;103(5):691–6. PubMed PMID: 10074486. Pubmed Central PMCID: 408131.

[76] Sakanaka M, Wen TC, Matsuda S, Masuda S, Morishita E, Nagao M, et al. In vivo evidence that erythropoietin protects neurons from ischemic damage. Proceedings of the national academy of sciences of the United States of America. 1998 Apr 14;95(8):4635–40. PubMed PMID: 9539790. Pubmed Central PMCID: 22542.

[77] Siren AL, Knerlich F, Poser W, Gleiter CH, Bruck W, Ehrenreich H. Erythropoietin and erythropoietin receptor in human ischemic/hypoxic brain. Acta neuropathologica. 2001 Mar;101(3):271–6. PubMed PMID: 11307627.

[78] Siren AL, Fratelli M, Brines M, Goemans C, Casagrande S, Lewczuk P, et al. Erythropoietin prevents neuronal apoptosis after cerebral ischemia and metabolic stress. Proceedings of the National Academy of Sciences of the United States of America. 2001 Mar 27;98(7):4044–9. PubMed PMID: 11259643. Pubmed Central PMCID: 31176.

[79] Soliz J, Joseph V, Soulage C, Becskei C, Vogel J, Pequignot JM, et al. Erythropoietin regulates hypoxic ventilation in mice by interacting with brainstem and carotid bodies. The journal of physiology. 2005 Oct 15;568(Pt 2):559–71. PubMed PMID: 16051624. Pubmed Central PMCID: 1474739.

[80] Soliz J, Gassmann M, Joseph V. Soluble erythropoietin receptor is present in the mouse brain and is required for the ventilatory acclimatization to hypoxia. The journal of physiology. 2007 Aug 15;583(Pt 1):329–36. PubMed PMID: 17584830. Pubmed Central PMCID: 2277219.

[81] Soliz J, Soulage C, Hermann DM, Gassmann M. Acute and chronic exposure to hypoxia alters ventilatory pattern but not minute ventilation of mice overexpressing erythropoietin. American journal of physiology regulatory, integrative and comparative physiology. 2007 Oct;293(4):R1702–10. PubMed PMID: 17652365.

[82] Weissmann N, Manz D, Buchspies D, Keller S, Mehling T, Voswinckel R, et al. Congenital erythropoietin over-expression causes "anti-pulmonary hypertensive" structural and functional changes in mice, both in normoxia and hypoxia. Thrombosis and haemostasis. 2005 Sep;94(3):630–8. PubMed PMID: 16268482.

[83] Ruifrok WP, de Boer RA, Westenbrink BD, van Veldhuisen DJ, van Gilst WH. Erythropoietin in cardiac disease: new features of an old drug. European journal of pharmacology. 2008 May 13;585(2–3):270–7. PubMed PMID: 18407263.

[84] Hagstrom L, Agbulut O, El-Hasnaoui-Saadani R, Marchant D, Favret F, Richalet JP, et al. Epo is relevant neither for microvascular formation nor for the new formation and maintenance of mice skeletal muscle fibres in both normoxia and hypoxia. Journal of biomedicine & biotechnology. 2010;2010:137817. PubMed PMID: 20414335. Pubmed Central PMCID: 2855079.

[85] Hagstrom L, Canon F, Agbulut O, Marchant D, Serrurier B, Richalet JP, et al. Skeletal muscle intrinsic functional properties are preserved in a model of erythropoietin deficient mice exposed to hypoxia. Pflugers archiv: European journal of physiology. 2010 Apr;459(5):713–23. PubMed PMID: 20119684.

[86] Pichon A, Lamarre Y, Voituron N, Marchant D, Vilar J, Richalet JP, et al. Red blood cell deformability is very slightly decreased in erythropoietin deficient mice. Clinical hemorheology and microcirculation. 2014;56(1):41–6. PubMed PMID: 23302595.

6

Epigenetic Programming of Cardiovascular Disease by Perinatal Hypoxia and Fetal Growth Restriction

Paola Casanello, Emilio A. Herrera and
Bernardo J. Krause

Abstract

Most of the worldwide deaths in patients with non-communicable diseases are due to cardiovascular and metabolic diseases, which are determined by a mix of environmental, genetic and epigenetic factors, and by their interactions. The aetiology of most cardiovascular diseases has been partially linked with *in utero* adverse conditions that may increase the risk of developing diseases later in life, known as Developmental Origins of Health and Disease (DOHaD). Perinatal hypoxia can program the fetal and postnatal developmental patterns, resulting in permanent modifications of cells, organs and systems function. In spite of the vast evidence obtained from human and animal studies linking development under adverse intrauterine conditions with increased cardiovascular risk, still few is known about the specific effects of intrauterine oxygen deficiency and the related pathogenic mechanisms. Currently, the most accepted processes that program cellular function are epigenetic mechanisms which determine gene expression in a cell-specific fashion. In this chapter we will review the current literature regarding the perinatal exposure to chronic hypoxia and Fetal Growth Restriction (FGR) in humans and animals and how this impinges the cardiovascular physiology through epigenetic, biochemical, morphologic and pathophysiologic modifications that translate into diseases blasting at postnatal life.

Keywords: hypoxia, programming, vascular function, oxidative stress, epigenetics, chronic diseases

1. Introduction

The worldwide prevalence of cardiovascular diseases (CVDs) and metabolic syndrome ranges between 20 and 40%. These figures are likely to rise over the next decades [1, 2]. Genetic changes associated with the traits of the metabolic syndrome and cardiovascular diseases are able to explain a small proportion of cases [3], suggesting the presence of other contributory factors in these conditions. Epidemiologic studies in the late 1980s in the UK revealed a strong correlation with perinatal and fetal growth patterns. Fetal growth restriction (FGR) is thus associated with an increased risk of developing adult cardiometabolic diseases [4]. Multiple reports from across the world have documented the association between intrauterine growth mediators in early life with lifelong health. These are now recognized to be important risks in the development of non-communicable diseases in adult life. This concept so-called "Fetal Programming" has evolved into "Developmental Origins of Health and Disease" (DOHaD), which we refer as Intrauterine Programming (IUP) [5] for the purpose of this chapter. The present efforts in this field are focused on unveiling the physiological and molecular mechanisms, which drive IUP, and exploring opportunities to prevent or revert the long-term consequences. The physiologic and biochemical changes that explain IUP relate to the timing and stage of development when the insult takes place; the earlier in development, the stronger the long-term effects [5]. Conversely, the long-term consequences of IUP and reproducibility of the related phenotypes suggest that epigenetic mechanisms may underlay the altered "cell programming" [6].

2. Fetal growth restriction

Fetal growth restriction (FGR) is clinically defined by a fetal weight below the 10th percentile of normal for gestational age, but in a generic manner, FGR is a condition in which the potential growth of the fetus is negatively influenced by environmental and maternal factors [7]. The short-term consequences of FGR are LBW and the corresponding phenotype, which is associated with increased perinatal morbidity and mortality [8]. The long-term effects include a two- to threefold increase in the risk of developing cardiovascular disease (hypertension and coronary heart disease) in adult life [9]. The higher CVD risk in adults resulting from FGR can be traced back to a reduced arterial compliance in pre-pubertal subjects [10] and a decreased peripheral endothelial-dependent vascular relaxation at birth [11]. Moreover, studies in human placentae show that FGR-related endothelial dysfunction can also be detected in chorionic and umbilical arteries [12, 13]. Notably, we have recently demonstrated the presence of functional and epigenetic markers of endothelial dysfunction in systemic and umbilical arteries from FGR guinea pigs. The presence of these comparable markers suggests that umbilical artery endothelial cells (ECs) may be useful to explore the endothelial function of the fetus. The etiology of FGR in humans is not fully understood; however, there are known maternal risk factors such as living at high altitude, malnutrition, smoking, stress, and vascular dysfunction [14] which induce placental dysfunction and consequently fetal growth restriction. Presently, oxygen, glucose, free radicals, amino acids, and hormones have been shown to play an important role in modulating fetal growth and development. These factors are dynamically regulated throughout gestation [15]. In the earlier stages, limitations in oxygen supply promote trophoblast proliferation; however, persistence in a hypoxic environment as occurs in FGR harms trophoblast invasion and the transformation of spiral arteries leading to a vascular dysfunction of the placenta and impaired fetal growth. Thus, chronic hypoxia and oxidative stress have an important role in the placental dysfunction observed in FGR [15]. Several studies on humans confirm the presence of molecular markers of oxidative stress in the FGR placentae, the fetus, and the mother [16–19]. Impaired placental vascular function has also been proposed to play a role in FGR, conditioned by augmented synthesis and response to vasoconstrictors [20] and limited action of vasodilators [13], as well as by an increased inhibition of endothelial-dependent relaxation mediated by prooxidants [21].

Appropriate maternal nutrient supply to the fetus is key for its development. Several approaches limiting maternal supply (i.e., diet restriction) and placental nutrient transfer have been used to alter the normal fetal growth rate and development. In order to address this issue, various animal models (sheep, rat, rabbit, and guinea pig) have been developed, where placental dysfunction is induced by a reduction in uterine blood flow [22, 23]. We have recently developed a novel model of FGR in guinea pigs, by a progressive bilateral occlusion of the uterine arteries during the second half of gestation that gradually alters placental vascular resistance [24]. Several aspects suggest that this model is relevant to human clinical significance. For instance, guinea pigs present a decreased fetal abdominal growth and impaired placental blood flow adaptation during gestation, with a preserved brain blood flow and development, translating into an asymmetric FGR. Additionally, higher resistance to blood flow in the umbilical arteries can be observed. These are relevant clinical markers of FGR. However, most of mammalian models that develop placental insufficiency present a mixed effect of undernutrition, hypoxia, and oxidative stress [22]. Therefore, complementary models on chick embryos have been used to isolate the unique fetal effects of hypoxia during development from maternal responses [22]. Interestingly, the follow-up of the chickens gestated under hypoxia has shown important insights into the pathophysiological mechanisms that impair the cardiovascular function. For instance, Tintu et al. showed that developmental hypoxia induces cardiomyopathy associated with left ventricular dilatation, reduced ventricular wall mass, and increased apoptosis [25]. These responses were coupled with pump dysfunction, decreased ejection fractions, and diastolic dysfunction, which persisted in adulthood. Further, Salinas et al. showed marked cardiovascular morphostructural changes in high-altitude chicks, which were reverted either by incubation at low altitude or by oxygen supplementation [26]. Notably, Herrera et al. followed up these chicks to adulthood describing cardiac impairment in the capacity to response to pressor challenges [27]. In addition to the cardiovascular system, several organs/functions are affected during developmental hypoxia such as central nervous system, lung, and systemic metabolism. As well as in mammalian physiology, it seems that oxidative stress might be key in establishing the impairments induced by developmental hypoxia [28].

2.1. Hypoxia and oxidative stress in FGR

Hypoxia is defined as a limited oxygen (O_2) supply relative to the physiological demands of a tissue, organ, or organism. This is a restrictive condition frequently seen in the hypobaric environment (hypoxia of high altitude) or by a diminished oxygen delivery. At lowlands, hypoxia is a restrictive condition often faced during fetal life, either by maternal, umbilical-placental, or fetal conditions. Placental insufficiency leads to fetal growth restriction due to a chronic decrease in fetoplacental perfusion. This situation affects simultaneously O_2 and nutrient supply to the fetus [29], overlapping conditions that become difficult to isolate in order to assess the specific effect of O_2 deficiency in determining vascular impairment. Using avian models of FGR has served to establish that chronic hypoxia, independent of nutrition, plays a crucial role in vascular programming [30, 31]. Studies of vascular function during fetal life show remarkable similarities between the effect of hypoxia in chick embryos and placental insufficiency in mammals [26, 28]; they have also served to assess the long-term consequences [27]. In both cases (chick embryos and mammalian fetuses), the presence of endothelial dysfunction and vascular remodeling is observed mainly in peripheral arteries. The mechanism by which hypoxia induces cell damage in either case is the result of an increased generation of reactive oxygen species (ROS) due to an incomplete reduction of oxygen [15, 32].

The imbalance between endogenous antioxidant defenses and reactive oxygen species, where ROS overwhelms the antioxidant capacity, has been termed "oxidative stress" [33]. ROS includes a wide variety of highly reactive molecules, such as superoxide anion ($\cdot O_2^-$), hydrogen peroxide (H_2O_2), $\cdot NO$, peroxynitrite (ONOO-), organic hydroperoxide (ROOH), hypochlorous acid (HOCl), and hydroxyl ($\cdot OH$), alkoxy ($RO\cdot$), and peroxy radicals ($ROO\cdot$) [34]. Superoxide is the main ROS acting at the vascular level; it derives from the enzymatic activity of NOX (NADPH oxidases), XOR (xanthine oxidases), mitochondrial complexes I and III, uncoupled eNOS, and iNOS. In the case of NOS, ROS generation can occur because of reduced L-arginine (substrate) or BH_4 (cofactor) availability [33], uncoupling eNOS enzymes. Consequently, NOS-derived $\cdot O_2^-$ rapidly reacts with NO generating ONOO-, which reduces NO levels and modifies the structure of proteins, lipids, and DNA, causing endothelial dysfunction. Thus, increased oxidative stress exerts a negative effect on eNOS activity and NO bioavailability at multiple levels [33].

In FGR, compelling data show that oxidative stress in parallel to chronic hypoxia contributes to vascular dysfunction in the mother, placenta, and fetus [14]. In fact, short-term hypoxia induces eNOS expression and activation in human umbilical artery endothelial cells (HUAECs) [35], while in FGR HUAEC, there is reduced eNOS activation [13]. Conversely, FGR subjects present at birth increased levels of lipid peroxidation and decreased the activity of antioxidant enzymes and circulating mediators [36]. Additionally, markers of oxidative stress have been positively associated with increased umbilical artery pulsatility index, particularly in pregnancies affected by FGR [37]. We recently addressed the role of oxidative stress in FGR by treating pregnant guinea pigs with N-acetyl cysteine, a glutathione precursor, during the second half of gestation. Our results show that maternal treatment with NAC restores fetal growth by increasing placental efficiency and reverses endothelial dysfunction in FGR guinea pigs [38]. Similarly, *in ovo* melatonin administration to chronic hypoxic chick embryos reduces the levels of oxidative stress markers (i.e., lipid peroxidation and protein nitration), by increasing the expression of glutathione peroxidase (GPx), an antioxidant enzyme [28]. This effect is associated with improved endothelial function and reversal of fetal hypoxia-induced vascular remodeling; however, melatonin does not prevent FGR. Even more, in a chronic hypoxic sheep model, melatonin decreased maternal oxidative stress but simultaneously enhanced fetal growth restriction [39]. In summary, these data suggest that hypoxia and oxidative stress participate in the genesis of FGR-induced vascular dysfunction.

However, there is a need for further studies addressing the precise molecular mechanisms and effective treatments for hypoxic FGR and IUP.

At a molecular level, transcription factors nuclear factor kappa B (NFκB) [34] and nuclear factor E2-related factor 2 (Nrf2) implicated in oxidative stress [34, 40] participate in promoting and reducing cellular oxidative stress, respectively. Interestingly, Nrf2 presents the suggested properties of an oxidative stress sensor. Nrf2 is normally bound to Keap1, which targets the complex to proteasome degradation; however, a prooxidant milieu induces the oxidation of two cysteine residues in Keap1 and the release of Nrf2 that subsequently translocate to the nucleus [34]. The antioxidant response triggered by Nrf2 includes the expression of NAD(P)H dehydrogenase quinone 1 (NQO1), heme-oxygenase (HO), and other antioxidant enzymes [40]. Studies show that Nrf2-induced expression of NQO1 and HO-1 improves endothelial dysfunction increasing eNOS efficiency. However, there is no information addressing whether changes in the expression of genes involved in the antioxidant defense are present in early stages of endothelial dysfunction in FGR and whether they can be modulated during gestation.

3. Epigenetics and endothelial programming in FGR

Alteration in fetal development and IUP results in permanent changes in the physiological responses to different stressors across the life course. Undoubtedly, this represents a potential "handicap" for long-term health. Growing evidence in humans from individuals with altered fetal growth, and from animal models associated with the development of later cardiometabolic alterations, confirms the presence of epigenetic markers in different cell types [41]. Epigenetics can be considered as "chromosome-based mechanisms that modify the phenotypic plasticity of a cell or organism" [6]. Development itself is controlled by epigenetic mechanisms, which regulate cell differentiation and record environmental signals under physiologic [42] and/or pathologic conditions [43]. These epigenetic mechanisms include DNA methylation, a plethora of histone posttranslational modifications (PTM) (acetylation, methylation, phosphorylation, and others), ATP-dependent chromatin modifications, and noncoding RNAs [44].

3.1. DNA methylation

In higher animals, DNA is methylated via an enzymatic activity that transfers a methyl group to the 5′ position of cytosine ring on CpG dinucleotide generating 5-methyl-cytosine, a reaction catalyzed by two different families of DNA methyltransferases (DNMTs), named DNMT1 and DNMT3 (DNMT3a and DNMT3b) encoded by three different genes [45]. The role of DNMT1 is to preserve the DNA methylation pattern after DNA replication during mitotic cell division as well as after fertilization [46], a process guided by the presence of hemi-methylated CpGs, which are recognized by DNMT1 in dsDNA [47]. Additionally, DNMT3a and DNMT3b catalyze *de novo* methylation allowing the establishment of new DNA methylation patterns during gametogenesis, embryonic development, and cell differentiation [46, 48]. Interestingly, the genome of different cell types from a single subject presents a high DNA methylation density;

however, larger differences occur in the promoter regions of genes representing less than 5% of the total genomic DNA methylation [49]. Nonetheless, these subtle differences are likely controlling most cell-specific proteins expression at the whole organism level [50]. It is commonly accepted that DNA methylation represents a hallmark of reduced gene expression and long-term gene silencing [51, 52]; however, it is worth noting that growing evidence suggests a more dynamic role for this mechanism in the regulation of gene expression [51].

3.2. Histone posttranslational modifications

The protein structural unit of the chromosomes, the nucleosome, is formed by two copies of four histones proteins named H2A, H2B, H3, and H4. Additionally, these proteins present a globular domain to interact with other histones, and a flexible tail that participates actively in the interaction with DNA. Unlike DNA methylation, histone posttranslational modifications (PTMs) are more dynamic and do not give a straight idea regarding gene silencing or activation [52]. Moreover, histone PTMs are closely related with the context in which they take place and the presence of additional PTMs, suggesting the existence of a "histone code." Up to date, more than 50 enzymes that catalyze diverse histone modifications have been identified and classified according to the reaction they carry out [53]. **Histone acetylation** occurs in lysine residues (K) and involves the transference of an acetyl group from acetyl-CoA. In mammals, this reaction is carried out by three families of histone acetyl-transferases (HAT) named GNAT, MYST, and CBP/p300 [54]. This modification is considered an activator of gene expression, due to the fact that it stabilizes the positive charge of the lysine in the histone, reducing its affinity for DNA, avoiding the formation of highly compacted chromatin. The best characterized acetylations are those that take place in lysine 9 (K9), K14, K18, and K56 in histone 3 (H3) and K5, K8, K13, and K16 in H4 [55]. At least four types of **histone deacetylases** (HDAC I, II, III y IV) have been identified, which catalyze the reverse reaction of that done by the **histone acetyl-transferase**. This enzymatic reaction is related to gene silencing, progression of cell cycle, differentiation, and the response induced by DNA damage [56]. HDAC activity can be induced in response to DNA methylation, once repressor proteins that bind CpGs (MCP) are recruited. The latter have a site of interaction with several HDACs, suggesting that gene silencing could result from a combined action of DNA and histone modifications [51, 57].

3.3. Noncoding RNAs

The idea that noncoding RNAs could regulate the expression of genes was first proposed in the early 1960s [58], with a substantial progress in this field during the last decade. Less than 5% of the transcribed RNA encodes proteins; thus, most of them correspond to noncoding RNAs (ncRNAs) involved mainly in the regulation of gene expression [59, 60]. "Long" ncRNA (lncRNA), small interfering RNA (siRNA), and micro-RNA (miRNA) are the main regulatory ncRNAs. The lncRNA regulates the expression of a specific gene complementary either through chromatin remodeling, alternative mRNA processing (splicing), or siRNA generation [59]. Conversely, siRNA and miRNAs are interference RNA-based epigenetic mechanisms, which silence genes via noncoding RNAs of ~21 bp. To date, more than a thousand noncoding miRNAs have been reported. These are transcribed by the RNA polymerase II and encoded by specific genes (~70%) or, in lesser amounts, within the intronic regions of gene encoding proteins. Micro-RNAs are transcribed as pre-miRNA and initially processed in the nucleus by the DROSHA-DGCR8 complex. Subsequently, they are exported to the cytoplasm for miRNA maturation by the action of the complex formed by the DICER1 protein and RNase IIIa IIIb [61]. This processing leads to a single-strand RNA, which is incorporated into the "protein-induced silencing complex miRNA" (miRISC), which binds to a complementary region in a target mRNA. It has been proposed that a full complementarity between the miRNA and mRNA leads to degradation of the mRNA, while partial complementarity suppresses translation [62]. Notably, a single miRNA can regulate the expression of multiple mRNAs often associated signaling pathways or metabolic processes, while several miRNAs may converge in the regulation of a single mRNA constituting a complex mechanism for gene expression regulation [61, 62].

3.4. Epigenetics in endothelial physiology

Vascular development and endothelial differentiation and function require a fine epigenetic tuning, suggesting that epigenetic mechanisms play a key role in the IUP-associated vascular dysfunction [6]. The first stages of vascular development are determined by genetic factors, while the next processes that take place (i.e., blood vessel structure, identity, and function) are influenced/determined by hemodynamic factors, ROS, and oxygen levels [63, 64]. Considering that the effect of endothelial-specific transcription factors such as KLF2 and HoxA9 does not explain the protein expression levels present in this cell type [65], an "endothelial epigenetic code" regulating the expression of crucial genes has been suggested [52, 66]. Growing evidence shows that DNA methylation, histone PTM, and miRNAs [67] play an important role in the embryonic origins of endothelial cells (EC), as well as their homeostasis during life. The epigenetic regulation of *NOS3* gene has been extensively studied in EC and non-EC, showing that ECs have a distinctive pattern of DNA methylation and histone PTMs [65]. Conversely, the decreased expression of eNOS in HUVEC exposed to acute hypoxia is controlled by the overexpression of a natural cis-antisense noncoding RNA called sONE [68] and changes in histone PTM which occur specifically at the promoter of eNOS [69]. Similarly, in the endothelium, hypoxia and oxidative stress regulate the expression of several miRNAs that modify the expression of eNOS and other enzymes related to its short- and long-term function [70]. In support of this notion, we have recently demonstrated that eNOS-induced NO enhances arginase-2 expression by epigenetic modifications in the histones residing at *ARG2* gene promoter [71]. In summary, these data show that EC-specific eNOS expression, as well as other genes related with the L-arginine/NO pathway, is effectively controlled by multiple epigenetic mechanisms which are strongly influenced by hypoxia.

3.5. Epigenetics and endothelial dysfunction

Diverse studies show that epigenetic mechanisms can increase the risk or directly participate in the development of vascular diseases. In humans, ECs from atherosclerotic plaques have decreased levels of estrogen receptor-β along with increased DNA methylation at the promoter region of this gene, compared with nonatherosclerotic plaques cells [72]. Further studies in mice [73] and swine [74] have demonstrated that disturbed flow induces genome-wide changes in the DNA methylation of EC in vivo and in vitro, an effect that would be dependent on DNMT1 expression and that mainly affects genes related to oxidative stress. Conversely, abrogation of *Nos3* promoter DNA methylation increases basal eNOS mRNA expression in vitro and protects against hind limb ischemia injury in vivo [75]. Similarly, growing evidence suggests a central role of miRNAs in the genesis of cardiometabolic dysfunction, also proposed as sensitive molecular markers of vascular disease [76]. In fact, we recently reported that circulating levels of miRNA Let-7 and miR-126 are associated with different traits of cardiometabolic dysfunction in children as well as have a predictive value for metabolic syndrome in these subjects [77]. Comparable results in adults with type 2 diabetes have been reported, where increased levels of miR-21 and decreased levels of miR-126 correlated with cardiovascular and inflammatory complications [78].

In the context of IUP of endothelial dysfunction in rats, it has been shown that brief exposure to hypoxia at the end of gestation induces pulmonary vascular dysfunction in the newborn, which associates with increased eNOS expression accompanied by decreased DNA methylation in *Nos3* gene promoter [79]. Similarly, we reported a few years ago for the first time the presence of an altered epigenetic programming of eNOS expression in EC derived from human umbilical arteries of FGR patients [12]. Notably, the altered expression of eNOS was reversed by silencing DNMT1 expression in FGR EC, which restored the DNA methylation pattern at *NOS3* promoter, as well as the regulation of eNOS expression induced by hypoxia [12]. Furthermore, using a guinea pig model of FGR, we compared the eNOS expression and DNA methylation pattern at *Nos3* promoter to clarify whether these epigenetic changes occurring in umbilical EC would represent changes that take place in systemic arteries (i.e., aorta and femoral) [38]. We found comparable changes in eNOS expression which were associated with specific changes in DNA methylation of *Nos3* promoter in the different FGR EC studied, suggesting the presence of a common programming of endothelial dysfunction in the umbilical-placental and systemic circulation. Of note, maternal treatment with an antioxidant (NAC) prevented this epigenetic programming, restoring the eNOS mRNA levels to values observed in control fetuses. Similar studies have shown the beneficial effects of antioxidants during development, showing clear evidences that ROS have causal roles in cardiovascular programming [32]. In addition, several authors have shown that ROS may induce important epigenetic modifications that determined cardiovascular dysfunction later in life. Hypoxia and oxidative stress have been shown to be present in several conditions during pregnancy, such as preeclampsia, placental insufficiency, and high-altitude pregnancies [80]. In addition, assisted reproductive technologies induce hypoxic conditions at very early stages of development. All of the above studies have suggested epigenetic modifications of the eNOS gene [80, 81]. Conversely, the response to hypoxia and oxidative stress is primarily mediated by the hypoxia-inducible transcription factor (HIF), which is regulated by the oxygen-sensing HIF hydroxylases, members of the 2-oxoglutarate (2OG)-dependent oxygenase family. Similarly, there are demethylases from the same family modulating methylation levels. Both systems, a transcription factor and an epigenetic regulator, are being regulated by hypoxia [82]. Further, HIF-1α has been suggested as an epigenetic modulator determining chromatin remodeling of hypoxia-responsive elements (HREs) sites [83]. Interestingly, in this report, a marked hyperacetylation of histones H3 and H4 was observed in the placental growth factor (Plgf) intron in hypoxic conditions. Further studies are needed to determine the interaction of transcription factors and epigenetic regulation, which might be an efficient way of controlling gene expression.

Another epigenetic regulatory mechanism is the miRNAs in the IUP. Present evidence suggests that miRNAs could be transferred across the placenta [84] with important consequences on fetal and maternal physiology. In humans, circulating levels of miR-21 during gestation in the mother positively correlate with evidence of fetal hypoxia [85] and evidence from in vitro studies show the participation of miR-21 in the FGR placental vascular dysfunction [86, 87]. By contrast, placental miR-126 levels negatively correlate with the FGR severity [88]. Studies in umbilical endothelium from swine fetuses have shown that the expression of miRNA that targets eNOS and VEGF pathways can be modulated by maternal supplementation with an L-arginine precursor [89]. Similarly, undernutrition decreases and programs at long term the expression of an anti-remodeling miRNA and this effect is prevented by the *in utero* inhibition of corticosteroid synthesis in pregnant rats [90].

4. Potential role of hypoxia-induced miRNAs, miR-21 and miR-126, on the endothelial dysfunction in FGR

As previously discussed, ncRNAs constitute an important epigenetic mechanism, which mainly regulates RNA translation; notably miR-21 and miR-126 represent two potential miR-NAs with a crucial role in the endothelium. In fact, both miRNAs are abundantly expressed in cultured endothelium [91] and respond to hypoxia with a substantial increase in miR-21 and miR-126 levels, representing ~40% of all the miRNAs present in this cell type [92]. In contrast to most miRNAs, miR-126 and miR-21 are encoded within the intronic region of genes coding for proteins. MiR-126 is encoded in the seventh intron of the gene for the endothelial-specific protein epidermal growth factor-like domain 7 (Egfl7) and its expression is partially (~30%) dependent on transcription factors that bind to the promoter region of this Egfl7 [93]. Additionally, miR-126 expression is regulated, independently of Egfl7, by the DNA methylation status of a miR-126-specific promoter located in intron 7 of Egfl7 [94], as well as the binding of Nrf2 to this region in response to oxidative stress [95]. Preliminary data from our group show that FGR human endothelial cells present increased levels of DNA methylation in miR-126 promoter, suggesting an epigenetic programming of this miRNA in FGR endothelium. Conversely, miR-21 is encoded in the 11th intron of the stress-induced protein TMEM49, but its expression is completely controlled by a specific promoter in the intron 10 of TMEM49 with predicted binding sites for transcription factors that respond to oxidative stress and inflammation [96, 97]. This suggests that the expression of miR-21 and miR-126 could be regulated by epigenetic modifications present in their specific intronic promoters.

It has been proposed that miR-126 is an endothelial-specific miRNA which promotes angiogenic activation in progenitor cells during early development, as well as vascular repair in adult subjects, while in mature endothelial cells, it has an anti-atherogenic effect maintaining endothelial quiescence and preventing inflammation [67]. In ob/ob mice, antioxidant treatment induces a miR-126-dependent anti-inflammatory and antioxidant vascular response [98], an effect also observed in HUVEC [99]. Both miRNAs, miR-21 and miR-126, are upregulated by unidirectional shear stress, protecting EC from apoptosis and increasing the activation of eNOS [100]. However, in oscillatory shear stress conditions, increased levels of miR-21 promote the expression of pro-inflammatory mediators [101]. Thus, it has been proposed that miR-21 has a dual effect on vascular function: over a short time, it protects against hypoxia and ischemia [70, 102–104], and over the longer term, leads to endothelial dysfunction, apoptosis [70, 102, 105, 106], and eNOS dysfunction. The latter would occur by targeting the expression of antioxidant enzymes [70], as well as enhancing the levels of the endogenous eNOS inhibitor asymmetric dimethyl arginine (ADMA) by downregulating the expression of the enzyme dimethyl arginine dimethylaminohydrolase 1 (DDAH1) [105, 107, 108]. These data suggest that the dynamic regulation of miR-21 and miR-126 could participate in the early defense of the endothelium to hypoxia and oxidative stress; nonetheless, they prime endothelial dysfunction over the long term. Thus, increased levels of miR-21 and decreased expression of miR-126 observed in FGR placentae at term could represent a consequence rather than a cause of the hypoxia-induced endothelial dysfunction.

5. Conclusions

The programming of vascular, particularly endothelial dysfunction by hypoxia in FGR is an important issue in fetal-maternal medicine up to date. Currently, there is a serious need to undercover the real impact of hypoxia as a driving force to perinatal and postnatal cardiovascular and metabolic diseases, pointing out the main proposed mechanisms. The reviewed data support the notion that epigenetic mechanisms contribute to defining and regulating vascular responses to pathological stimuli (leading to FGR). However, evidence of how fetal exposure to hypoxia and oxidative stress lead to epigenetic modifications remains elusive.

Therefore, new knowledge on the role of epigenetic mechanisms involved in the long-term vascular function is crucial to understand and put into context adequate interventions. The timing of the vascular adaptations and epigenetic responses is one of the most relevant questions that need to be answered in order to prioritize clinical approaches to early diagnose and treat such perinatal conditions, limiting postnatal cardiometabolic risk in the progeny.

Author details

Paola Casanello[1, 2]*, Emilio A. Herrera[3] and Bernardo J. Krause[1]

*Address all correspondence to: paolacasanello@gmail.com

1 Division of Pediatrics, Department of Neonatology, The Pontifical Catholic University of Chile, Santiago, Chile

2 Division of Obstetrics & Gynecology, School of Medicine, The Pontifical Catholic University of Chile, Santiago, Chile

3 Pathophysiology Program, Biomedical Sciences Institute (ICBM), Faculty of Medicine, University of Chile, Santiago, Chile

References

[1] Alberti KG, Eckel RH, Grundy SM, Zimmet PZ, Cleeman JI, Donato KA, Fruchart JC, James WP, Loria CM, Smith SC, Jr.: Harmonizing the metabolic syndrome: a joint interim statement of the International Diabetes Federation Task Force on Epidemiology and Prevention; National Heart, Lung, and Blood Institute; American Heart Association; World Heart Federation; International Atherosclerosis Society; and International Association for the Study of Obesity. Circulation 2009, 120:1640–5.

[2] Escobedo J, Schargrodsky H, Champagne B, Silva H, Boissonnet CP, Vinueza R, Torres M, Hernandez R, Wilson E: Prevalence of the metabolic syndrome in Latin America and its association with sub-clinical carotid atherosclerosis: the CARMELA cross sectional study. Cardiovasc Diabetol 2009, 8:52.

[3] El Shamieh S, Visvikis-Siest S: Genetic biomarkers of hypertension and future challenges integrating epigenomics. Clin Chim Acta 2012, 414:259–65.

[4] Barker DJ: Birth weight and hypertension. Hypertension 2006, 48:357–8.

[5] Hanson MA, Gluckman PD: Early developmental conditioning of later health and disease: physiology or pathophysiology? Physiol Rev 2014, 94:1027–76.

[6] Krause B, Sobrevia L, Casanello P: Epigenetics: new concepts of old phenomena in vascular physiology. Curr Vasc Pharmacol 2009, 7:513–20.

[7] Zhang J, Merialdi M, Platt LD, Kramer MS: Defining normal and abnormal fetal growth: promises and challenges. Am J Obstet Gynecol 2010, 202:522–8.

[8] Romo A, Carceller R, Tobajas J: Intrauterine growth retardation (IUGR): epidemiology and etiology. Pediatr Endocrinol Rev 2009, 6(Suppl 3):332–6.

[9]   Cohen E, Wong FY, Horne RS, Yiallourou SR: Intrauterine growth restriction: impact on cardiovascular development and function throughout infancy. Pediatr Res 2016; 79(6):821–30.

[10] Martin H, Hu J, Gennser G, Norman M: Impaired endothelial function and increased carotid stiffness in 9-year-old children with low birthweight. Circulation 2000, 102:2739–44.

[11] Martin H, Gazelius B, Norman M: Impaired acetylcholine-induced vascular relaxation in low birth weight infants: implications for adult hypertension? Pediatr Res 2000, 47:457–62.

[12] Krause BJ, Costello PM, Munoz-Urrutia E, Lillycrop KA, Hanson MA, Casanello P: Role of DNA methyltransferase 1 on the altered eNOS expression in human umbilical endothelium from intrauterine growth restricted fetuses. Epigenetics: Official Journal of the DNA Methylation Society 2013, 8:944–52.

[13] Krause BJ, Carrasco-Wong I, Caniuguir A, Carvajal J, Farias M, Casanello P: Endothelial eNOS/arginase imbalance contributes to vascular dysfunction in IUGR umbilical and placental vessels. Placenta 2013, 34:20–8.

[14] Roberts JM: Pathophysiology of ischemic placental disease. Semin Perinatol 2014, 38:139–45.

[15] Herrera EA, Krause B, Ebensperger G, Reyes RV, Casanello P, Parra-Cordero M, Llanos AJ: The placental pursuit for an adequate oxidant balance between the mother and the fetus. Frontiers Pharmacol 2014, 5:149.

[16] Takagi Y, Nikaido T, Toki T, Kita N, Kanai M, Ashida T, Ohira S, Konishi I: Levels of oxidative stress and redox-related molecules in the placenta in preeclampsia and fetal growth restriction. Virchows Archiv: Int J Pathol 2004, 444:49–55.

[17] Biri A, Bozkurt N, Turp A, Kavutcu M, Himmetoglu O, Durak I: Role of oxidative stress in intrauterine growth restriction. Gynecol Obstet Invest 2007, 64:187–92.

[18] Bar-Or D, Heyborne KD, Bar-Or R, Rael LT, Winkler JV, Navot D: Cysteinylation of maternal plasma albumin and its association with intrauterine growth restriction. Prenatal Diag 2005, 25:245–9.

[19] Potdar N, Singh R, Mistry V, Evans MD, Farmer PB, Konje JC, Cooke MS: First-trimester increase in oxidative stress and risk of small-for-gestational-age fetus. Bjog 2009, 116:637–42.

[20] Wareing M, Greenwood SL, Fyfe GK, Baker PN: Reactivity of human placental chorionic plate vessels from pregnancies complicated by intrauterine growth restriction (IUGR). Biol Reprod 2006, 75:518–23.

[21] Schneider D, Hernandez C, Farias M, Uauy R, Krause BJ, Casanello P: Oxidative stress as common trait of endothelial dysfunction in chorionic arteries from fetuses with IUGR and LGA. Placenta 2015, 36:552–8.

[22] Swanson AM, David AL: Animal models of fetal growth restriction: Considerations for translational medicine. Placenta 2015, 36:623–30.

[23] Carter AM: Animal models of human placentation--a review. Placenta 2007, 28(Suppl A):S41–7.

[24] Herrera EA, Alegria R, Farias M, Diaz-Lopez F, Hernandez C, Uauy R, Regnault TR, Casanello P, Krause BJ: Assessment of in vivo fetal growth and placental vascular function in a novel intrauterine growth restriction model of progressive uterine artery occlusion in guinea pigs. J Physiol 2016, 594:1553–61.

[25] Tintu AN, Noble FA, Rouwet EV: Hypoxia disturbs fetal hemodynamics and growth. Endothelium 2007, 14:353–60.

[26] Salinas CE, Blanco CE, Villena M, Camm EJ, Tuckett JD, Weerakkody RA, Kane AD, Shelley AM, Wooding FB, Quy M, Giussani DA: Cardiac and vascular disease prior to hatching in chick embryos incubated at high altitude. J Dev Orig Health Dis 2010, 1:60–6.

[27] Herrera EA, Salinas CE, Blanco CE, Villena M, Giussani DA: High altitude hypoxia and blood pressure dysregulation in adult chickens. J Dev Origins Health Dis 2013, 4:69–76.

[28] Itani N, Skeffington KL, Beck C, Niu YG, Giussani DA: Melatonin rescues cardiovascular dysfunction during hypoxic development in the chick embryo. J Pineal Res 2016, 60:16–26.

[29] Marsal K: Obstetric management of intrauterine growth restriction. Best Pract Res Clin Obstet Gynaecol 2009, 23:857–70.

[30] Giussani DA, Salinas CE, Villena M, Blanco CE: The role of oxygen in prenatal growth: studies in the chick embryo. J Physiol Lond 2007, 585:911–7.

[31] Miller SL, Green LR, Peebles DM, Hanson MA, Blanco CE: Effects of chronic hypoxia and protein malnutrition on growth in the developing chick. Am J Obstet Gynecol 2002, 186:261–7.

[32] Giussani DA, Camm EJ, Niu Y, Richter HG, Blanco CE, Gottschalk R, Blake EZ, Horder KA, Thakor AS, Hansell JA, Kane AD, Wooding FB, Cross CM, Herrera EA: Developmental programming of cardiovascular dysfunction by prenatal hypoxia and oxidative stress. PLoS One 2012, 7:e31017.

[33] Forstermann U: Nitric oxide and oxidative stress in vascular disease. Pflugers Arch 2010, 459:923–39.

[34] Brigelius-Flohe R, Flohe L: Basic principles and emerging concepts in the redox control of transcription factors. Antioxid Redox Signal 2011, 15:2335–81.

[35] Krause BJ, Prieto CP, Munoz-Urrutia E, San Martin S, Sobrevia L, Casanello P: Role of arginase-2 and eNOS in the differential vascular reactivity and hypoxia-induced endothelial response in umbilical arteries and veins. Placenta 2012, 33:360–6.

[36] Leduc L, Delvin E, Ouellet A, Garofalo C, Grenierd E, Morin L, Dube J, Bouity-Voubou M, Moutquin JM, Fouron JC, Klam S, Levy E: Oxidized low-density lipoproteins in cord blood from neonates with intra-uterine growth restriction. Eur J Obst Gynecol Rep Biol 2011, 156:46–9.

[37] Guven ESG, Karcaaltincaba D, Kandemir O, Kiykac S, Mentese A: Cord blood oxidative stress markers correlate with umbilical artery pulsatility in fetal growth restriction. J Matern-Fetal Neo M 2013, 26:576–80.

[38] Herrera EA, Cifuentes-Zuniga F, Figueroa E, Villanueva C, Hernandez C, Alegria R, Arroyo V, Penaloza E, Farias M, Uauy R, Casanello P, Krause BJ: N-acetyl cysteine, a glutathione precursor, reverts vascular dysfunction and endothelial epigenetic programming in intrauterine growth restricted guinea pigs. J Physiol 2016, doi: 10.1113/JP273396

[39] Gonzalez-Candia A, Veliz M, Araya C, Quezada S, Ebensperger G, Seron-Ferre M, Reyes RV, Llanos AJ, Herrera EA: Potential adverse effects of antenatal melatonin as a treatment for intrauterine growth restriction: findings in pregnant sheep. Am J Obstet Gynecol 2016, 215:245 e1–7.

[40] McSweeney SR, Warabi E, Siow RC: Nrf2 as an endothelial mechanosensitive transcription factor: going with the flow. Hypertension 2016, 67:20–9.

[41] Hanson M, Godfrey KM, Lillycrop KA, Burdge GC, Gluckman PD: Developmental plasticity and developmental origins of non-communicable disease: Theoretical considerations and epigenetic mechanisms. Prog Biophys Mol Biol 2011, 106:272–80.

[42] Ohtani K, Dimmeler S: Epigenetic regulation of cardiovascular differentiation. Cardiovasc Res 2011, 90:404–12.

[43] Ordovas JM, Smith CE: Epigenetics and cardiovascular disease. Nat Rev Cardiol 2010, 7:510–9.

[44] Kim JK, Samaranayake M, Pradhan S: Epigenetic mechanisms in mammals. Cell Mol Life Sci 2009, 66:596–612.

[45] Goll MG, Bestor TH: Eukaryotic cytosine methyltransferases. Annu Rev Biochem 2005, 74:481–514.

[46] Reik W: Stability and flexibility of epigenetic gene regulation in mammalian development. Nature 2007, 447:425–32.

[47] Buryanov YI, Shevchuk TV: DNA methyltransferases and structural-functional specificity of eukaryotic DNA modification. Biochemistry (Mosc) 2005, 70:730–42.

[48] Collas P, Noer A, Timoskainen S: Programming the genome in embryonic and somatic stem cells. J Cell Mol Med 2007, 11:602–20.

[49] Suzuki MM, Bird A: DNA methylation landscapes: provocative insights from epigenomics. Nat Rev Genet 2008, 9:465–76.

[50] Illingworth RS, Bird AP: CpG islands – 'a rough guide'. FEBS Lett 2009, 583:1713–20.

[51] Klose RJ, Bird AP: Genomic DNA methylation: the mark and its mediators. Trends Biochem Sci 2006, 31:89–97.

[52] Kimura A, Matsubara K, Horikoshi M: A decade of histone acetylation: marking eukaryotic chromosomes with specific codes. J Biochem 2005, 138:647–62.

[53] Jenuwein T, Allis CD: Translating the histone code. Science 2001, 293:1074–80.

[54] Wang GG, Allis CD, Chi P: Chromatin remodeling and cancer, Part I: covalent histone modifications. Trends Mol Med 2007, 13:363–72.

[55] Berger SL: The complex language of chromatin regulation during transcription. Nature 2007, 447:407–12.

[56] Thiagalingam S, Cheng KH, Lee HJ, Mineva N, Thiagalingam A, Ponte JF: Histone deacetylases: unique players in shaping the epigenetic histone code. Ann N Y Acad Sci 2003, 983:84–100.

[57] Matouk CC, Marsden PA: Epigenetic regulation of vascular endothelial gene expression. Circ Res 2008, 102:873–87.

[58] Britten RJ, Davidson EH: Gene regulation for higher cells: a theory. Science 1969, 165:349–57.

[59] Kaikkonen MU, Lam MT, Glass CK: Non-coding RNAs as regulators of gene expression and epigenetics. Cardiovasc Res 2011, 90:430–40.

[60] Deng K, Wang H, Guo X, Xia J: The cross talk between long, non-coding RNAs and microRNAs in gastric cancer. Acta Biochim Biophys Sin 2016;48(2):111–6.

[61] Lin S, Gregory RI: MicroRNA biogenesis pathways in cancer. Nat Rev Cancer 2015, 15:321–33.

[62] Afonso-Grunz F, Muller S: Principles of miRNA-mRNA interactions: beyond sequence complementarity. Cell Mol Life Sci 2015, 72:3127–41.

[63] le Noble F, Klein C, Tintu A, Pries A, Buschmann I: Neural guidance molecules, tip cells, and mechanical factors in vascular development. Cardiovasc Res 2008, 78:232–41.

[64] Ribatti D, Nico B, Crivellato E: Morphological and molecular aspects of physiological vascular morphogenesis. Angiogenesis 2009, 12:101–11.

[65] Fish JE, Marsden PA: Endothelial nitric oxide synthase: insight into cell-specific gene regulation in the vascular endothelium. Cell Mol Life Sci 2006, 63:144–62.

[66] Illi B, Colussi C, Rosati J, Spallotta F, Nanni S, Farsetti A, Capogrossi MC, Gaetano C: NO points to epigenetics in vascular development. Cardiovasc Res 2011, 90:447–56.

[67] Chistiakov DA, Orekhov AN, Bobryshev YV: The role of miR-126 in embryonic angiogenesis, adult vascular homeostasis, and vascular repair and its alterations in atherosclerotic disease. J Mol Cell Cardiol 2016, 97:47–55.

[68] Fish JE, Matouk CC, Yeboah E, Bevan SC, Khan M, Patil K, Ohh M, Marsden PA: Hypoxia-inducible expression of a natural cis-antisense transcript inhibits endothelial nitric-oxide synthase. J Biol Chem 2007, 282:15652–66.

[69] Fish JE, Yan MS, Matouk CC, St Bernard R, Ho JJ, Gavryushova A, Srivastava D, Marsden PA: Hypoxic repression of endothelial nitric-oxide synthase transcription is coupled with eviction of promoter histones. J Biol Chem 2010, 285:810–26.

[70] Marin T, Gongol B, Chen Z, Woo B, Subramaniam S, Chien S, Shyy JY: Mechanosensitive microRNAs-role in endothelial responses to shear stress and redox state. Free Radic Biol Med 2013, 64:61–8.

[71] Krause BJ, Hernandez C, Caniuguir A, Vasquez-Devaud P, Carrasco-Wong I, Uauy R, Casanello P: Arginase-2 is cooperatively up-regulated by nitric oxide and histone deacetylase inhibition in human umbilical artery endothelial cells. Biochem Pharmacol 2016, 99:53–9.

[72] Kim J, Kim JY, Song KS, Lee YH, Seo JS, Jelinek J, Goldschmidt-Clermont PJ, Issa JP: Epigenetic changes in estrogen receptor beta gene in atherosclerotic cardiovascular tissues and in-vitro vascular senescence. Biochim Biophys Acta 2007, 1772:72–80.

[73] Dunn J, Qiu H, Kim S, Jjingo D, Hoffman R, Kim CW, Jang I, Son DJ, Kim D, Pan C, Fan Y, Jordan IK, Jo H: Flow-dependent epigenetic DNA methylation regulates endothelial gene expression and atherosclerosis. J Clin Invest 2014, 124:3187–99.

[74] Jiang YZ, Manduchi E, Stoeckert CJ, Jr., Davies PF: Arterial endothelial methylome: differential DNA methylation in athero-susceptible disturbed flow regions in vivo. BMC Gen 2015, 16:506.

[75] Rao X, Zhong J, Zhang S, Zhang Y, Yu Q, Yang P, Wang MH, Fulton DJ, Shi H, Dong Z, Wang D, Wang CY: Loss of methyl-CpG-binding domain protein 2 enhances endothelial angiogenesis and protects mice against hind-limb ischemic injury. Circulation 2011, 123:2964–74.

[76] Navickas R, Gal D, Laucevicius A, Taparauskaite A, Zdanyte M, Holvoet P: Identifying circulating microRNAs as biomarkers of cardiovascular disease: a systematic review. Cardiovasc Res 2016.

[77] Krause BJ, Carrasco-Wong I, Dominguez A, Arnaiz P, Farias M, Barja S, Mardones F, Casanello P: Micro-RNAs Let7e and 126 in plasma as markers of metabolic dysfunction in 10 to 12 years old children. PLoS One 2015, 10:e0128140.

[78] Olivieri F, Spazzafumo L, Bonafe M, Recchioni R, Prattichizzo F, Marcheselli F, Micolucci L, Mensa E, Giuliani A, Santini G, Gobbi M, Lazzarini R, Boemi M, Testa R, Antonicelli R, Procopio AD, Bonfigli AR: MiR-21-5p and miR-126a-3p levels in plasma and circulating angiogenic cells: relationship with type 2 diabetes complications. Oncotarget 2015, 6:35372–82.

[79] Xu XF, Ma XL, Shen Z, Wu XL, Cheng F, Du LZ: Epigenetic regulation of the endothelial nitric oxide synthase gene in persistent pulmonary hypertension of the newborn rat. J Hypertens 2010, 28:2227–35.

[80] Sartori C, Rimoldi SF, Rexhaj E, Allemann Y, Scherrer U: Epigenetics in cardiovascular regulation. Adv Exp Med Biol 2016, 903:55–62.

[81] Rexhaj E, Paoloni-Giacobino A, Rimoldi SF, Fuster DG, Anderegg M, Somm E, Bouillet E, Allemann Y, Sartori C, Scherrer U: Mice generated by in vitro fertilization exhibit vascular dysfunction and shortened life span. J Clin Invest 2013, 123:5052–60.

[82] Hancock RL, Dunne K, Walport LJ, Flashman E, Kawamura A: Epigenetic regulation by histone demethylases in hypoxia. Epigenomics 2015, 7:791–811.

[83] Tudisco L, Della Ragione F, Tarallo V, Apicella I, D'Esposito M, Matarazzo MR, De Falco S: Epigenetic control of hypoxia inducible factor-1alpha-dependent expression of placental growth factor in hypoxic conditions. Epigen Off J DNA Meth Soc 2014, 9:600–10.

[84] Li J, Zhang Y, Li D, Liu Y, Chu D, Jiang X, Hou D, Zen K, Zhang CY: Small non-coding RNAs transfer through mammalian placenta and directly regulate fetal gene expression. Protein Cell 2015, 6:391–6.

[85] Whitehead CL, Teh WT, Walker SP, Leung C, Larmour L, Tong S: Circulating MicroRNAs in maternal blood as potential biomarkers for fetal hypoxia in-utero. PLoS One 2013, 8:e78487.

[86] Cindrova-Davies T, Herrera EA, Niu Y, Kingdom J, Giussani DA, Burton GJ: Reduced cystathionine gamma-lyase and increased miR-21 expression are associated with increased vascular resistance in growth-restricted pregnancies: hydrogen sulfide as a placental vasodilator. Am J Pathol 2013, 182:1448–58.

[87] Maccani MA, Padbury JF, Marsit CJ: miR-16 and miR-21 expression in the placenta is associated with fetal growth. PLoS One 2011, 6:e21210.

[88] Hromadnikova I, Kotlabova K, Hympanova L, Krofta L: Cardiovascular and cerebrovascular disease associated microRNAs are dysregulated in placental tissues affected with gestational hypertension, preeclampsia and intrauterine growth restriction. PLoS One 2015, 10:e0138383.

[89] Liu XD, Wu X, Yin YL, Liu YQ, Geng MM, Yang HS, Blachier F, Wu GY: Effects of dietary L-arginine or N-carbamylglutamate supplementation during late gestation of sows on the miR-15b/16, miR-221/222, VEGFA and eNOS expression in umbilical vein. Amino Acids 2012, 42:2111–9.

[90] Khorram O, Chuang TD, Pearce WJ: Long-term effects of maternal undernutrition on offspring carotid artery remodeling: role of miR-29c. J Dev Orig Health Dis 2015, 6:342–9.

[91] Guduric-Fuchs J, O'Connor A, Cullen A, Harwood L, Medina RJ, O'Neill CL, Stitt AW, Curtis TM, Simpson DA: Deep sequencing reveals predominant expression of miR-21 amongst the small non-coding RNAs in retinal microvascular endothelial cells. J Cell Biochem 2012, 113:2098–111.

[92] Voellenkle C, Rooij J, Guffanti A, Brini E, Fasanaro P, Isaia E, Croft L, David M, Capogrossi MC, Moles A, Felsani A, Martelli F: Deep-sequencing of endothelial cells exposed to hypoxia reveals the complexity of known and novel microRNAs. RNA 2012, 18:472–84.

[93] Harris TA, Yamakuchi M, Kondo M, Oettgen P, Lowenstein CJ: Ets-1 and Ets-2 regulate the expression of microRNA-126 in endothelial cells. Arterioscler Thromb Vasc Biol 2010, 30:1990–7.

[94] Watanabe K, Emoto N, Hamano E, Sunohara M, Kawakami M, Kage H, Kitano K, Nakajima J, Goto A, Fukayama M, Nagase T, Yatomi Y, Ohishi N, Takai D: Genome structure-based screening identified epigenetically silenced microRNA associated with invasiveness in non-small-cell lung cancer. Int J Cancer 2012, 130:2580–90.

[95] Kuosmanen SM, Viitala S, Laitinen T, Perakyla M, Polonen P, Kansanen E, Leinonen H, Raju S, Wienecke-Baldacchino A, Narvanen A, Poso A, Heinaniemi M, Heikkinen S, Levonen AL: The effects of sequence variation on genome-wide NRF2 binding – new target genes and regulatory SNPs. Nucl Acid Res 2016, 44:1760–75.

[96] Ribas J, Lupold SE: The transcriptional regulation of miR-21, its multiple transcripts, and their implication in prostate cancer. Cell Cycle 2010, 9:923–9.

[97] Kumarswamy R, Volkmann I, Thum T: Regulation and function of miRNA-21 in health and disease. RNA Biol 2011, 8:706–13.

[98] Togliatto G, Trombetta A, Dentelli P, Gallo S, Rosso A, Cotogni P, Granata R, Falcioni R, Delale T, Ghigo E, Brizzi MF: Unacylated ghrelin induces oxidative stress resistance in a glucose intolerance and peripheral artery disease mouse model by restoring endothelial cell miR-126 expression. Diabetes 2015, 64:1370–82.

[99] Sui XQ, Xu ZM, Xie MB, Pei DA: Resveratrol inhibits hydrogen peroxide-induced apoptosis in endothelial cells via the activation of PI3K/Akt by miR-126. J Atheroscler Thromb 2014, 21:108–18.

[100] Weber M, Baker MB, Moore JP, Searles CD: MiR-21 is induced in endothelial cells by shear stress and modulates apoptosis and eNOS activity. Biochem Biophys Res Commun 2010, 393:643–8.

[101] Zhou J, Wang KC, Wu W, Subramaniam S, Shyy JY, Chiu JJ, Li JY, Chien S. MicroRNA-21 targets peroxisome proliferators-activated receptor-{alpha} in an autoregulatory loop to modulate flow-induced endothelial inflammation. Proc Natl Acad Sci U S A 2011;108(25):10355-60.

[102] Xu X, Kriegel AJ, Jiao X, Liu H, Bai X, Olson J, Liang M, Ding X: miR-21 in ischemia/ reperfusion injury: a double-edged sword? Physiol Gen 2014, 46:789–97.

[103] Ge X, Han Z, Chen F, Wang H, Zhang B, Jiang R, Lei P, Zhang J: MiR-21 alleviates secondary blood-brain barrier damage after traumatic brain injury in rats. Brain Res 2015, 1603:150–7.

[104] Qiao S, Olson JM, Paterson M, Yan Y, Zaja I, Liu Y, Riess ML, Kersten JR, Liang M, Warltier DC, Bosnjak ZJ, Ge ZD: MicroRNA-21 Mediates isoflurane-induced cardio-protection against ischemia-reperfusion injury via Akt/nitric oxide synthase/mitochon-drial permeability transition pore pathway. Anesthesiology 2015, 123:786–98.

[105] Iannone L, Zhao L, Dubois O, Duluc L, Rhodes CJ, Wharton J, Wilkins MR, Leiper J, Wojciak-Stothard B: miR-21/DDAH1 pathway regulates pulmonary vascular responses to hypoxia. Biochem J 2014, 462:103–12.

[106] White K, Dempsie Y, Caruso P, Wallace E, McDonald RA, Stevens H, Hatley ME, Van Rooij E, Morrell NW, MacLean MR, Baker AH: Endothelial apoptosis in pulmonary hypertension is controlled by a microRNA/programmed cell death 4/caspase-3 axis. Hypertension 2014, 64:185–94.

[107] Chen L, Zhou JP, Kuang DB, Tang J, Li YJ, Chen XP: 4-HNE increases intracellular ADMA levels in cultured HUVECs: evidence for miR-21-dependent mechanisms. PLoS One 2013, 8:e64148.

[108] Zhao C, Li T, Han B, Yue W, Shi L, Wang H, Guo Y, Lu Z: DDAH1 deficiency promotes intracellular oxidative stress and cell apoptosis via a miR-21-dependent pathway in mouse embryonic fibroblasts. Free Radic Biol Med 2016, 92:50–60.

7

Hypoxic Upregulation of ARNT (HIF-1β): A Cell-Specific Attribute with Clinical Implications

Markus Mandl and Reinhard Depping

Abstract

According to the current point of view described in the literature, the transcription factor aryl hydrocarbon receptor nuclear translocator (ARNT), also designated as hypoxia-inducible factor (HIF)-1β, is constitutively expressed and not influenced by oxygen tension. However, a study published two decades ago provided early evidence regarding a hypoxia-dependent ARNT upregulation. This finding was subsequently challenged and neglected. Until now, only a limited number of publications focus on the regulation of ARNT in hypoxia. Therefore, appropriate studies and the putative mechanism mediating this cellular attribute are discussed. The advantages of an elevated ARNT expression level in tumour cells are delineated. This chapter provides an overview of hypoxia-inducible ARNT as an emerging concept in HIF biology.

Keywords: aryl hydrocarbon receptor nuclear translocator, ARNT, HIF-1β, crosstalk, cancer

1. Introduction

The name aryl hydrocarbon receptor nuclear translocator (ARNT) designates a transcription factor of the Per-ARNT-Sim family which is ubiquitously expressed. This protein is also known as hypoxia-inducible factor (HIF)-1β. The use of these two equal synonyms for the same transcription factor throughout the literature already implies its role in various signalling pathways [1]. Unfortunately, the term "hypoxia-inducible" might be misleading in this context. According to the current point of view described in the literature, ARNT expression is not affected by environmental conditions such as hypoxia. Therefore, ARNT is considered to be a constitutively expressed gene [1]. Although this notion might be true for the majority of cells/tissues investigated, numerous studies reported the capability of tumour cells to elevate

ARNT expression in response to hypoxia [1–7]. This cellular attribute was found in cells of different tumour types of both human and murine origin. These key findings clearly suggest that hypoxia-dependent ARNT upregulation might provide a certain benefit for appropriate cells [1].

ARNT and its paralogue ARNT2 [1] share a 90% identical amino acid sequence [8]. In contrast to ARNT, ARNT2 is mainly expressed in the central nervous system [8, 9]. ARNT2 expression was shown to be positively correlated with breast cancer prognosis [8]. In addition, high-ARNT2 levels in hepatocellular carcinomas are associated with a prolonged overall survival of cancer patients [8]. However, many functions of this transcription factor are still unknown [1, 8]. Moreover, the regulation of ARNT and ARNT2 varied in human hepatocellular carcinoma Hep3B cells. ARNT was elevated in hypoxia, whereas ARNT2 was not affected in this model [3].

This chapter describes the current knowledge regarding hypoxic upregulation of ARNT, which appears to be beneficial for certain types of tumour cells. Therefore, the aim of this section is to emphasise this unique cellular attribute. A potential altered ARNT expression level due to hypoxic exposure of cells should be considered and not generally excluded. In this context, the use of ARNT as loading control or as a reference gene is basically not recommended [1].

2. Regulation of ARNT

2.1. Upregulation of ARNT in response to hypoxia

First evidence for a hypoxia-dependent regulation of ARNT was provided by Wang et al. [5]. Herein, Hep3B cells were used to study the effects of HIF-1α and ARNT under hypoxic conditions. ARNT was elevated on mRNA level in this cell line due to hypoxic exposure (1% v/v O_2). In addition, treatment with hypoxia mimetics such as cobalt chloride and desferrioxamine had similar effects. Nuclear extracts prepared from Hep3B and HeLa cells were used to investigate the response of both HIF-1 subunits to oxygen deprivation. Re-oxygenation experiments were also included into the study [5]. The data revealed that both transcription factors HIF-1α and ARNT were inducible in hypoxic cells on mRNA as well as protein levels [5]. Huang et al. [10] reported that ARNT protein levels remained constant regardless of cellular oxygen tension. In this study, Hep3B, HeLa and HEK293 cells were used. Unfortunately, not all experiments were conducted with all cell lines [10], thereby making a direct comparison with the study of Wang et al. [5] complicated. Nevertheless, the latter report [10] challenged the results of the previous one [5] due to signal variations of Northern blots and discontinuities of time-course experiments [10].

However, Huang et al. [10] proposed a very graphic working model including a specific sensor for hypoxia located in the cell membrane [10]. The depicted mechanism is similar to our nowadays HIF scheme. These days the prolylhydroxylase domain enzymes (PHDs), which require O_2 as a substrate, are known to act as cellular oxygen sensors [11]. The comparison of both seminal studies conducted by Wang et al. [5] and Huang et al. [10] also requires a glance on citation frequencies of both reports. Noteworthily, the report of Wang et al. [5], which describes the upregulation of ARNT for the first time, was cited approximately four times more often as compared to Huang et al. [10]. Despite this clear distinction of citation frequencies, the opinion that ARNT is unaffected by cellular oxygen tension became a guideline in HIF biology [1].

The capability to elevate ARNT expression in hypoxia was also found in murine L929 and Hepa1 cells. Interestingly, human Hep3B cells were also used in this study conducted by Chilov et al. [7], but ARNT was unaffected by oxygen deprivation [7]. This seemingly conflicting observation compared to a previous report [5] is likely due to different experimental conditions. Obviously, a short-term exposure of Hep3B cells to hypoxia (4 h in Ref. [7]) is not sufficient to induce ARNT protein expression in this model. However, other studies clearly confirmed the hypoxia-dependent upregulation of ARNT in Hep3B cells [3, 4].

First mechanistic clues regarding the induction of ARNT under oxygen deprivation were provided by Zhong et al. [6]. Herein, the authors tested the hypothesis whether HIF-1α and ARNT are regulated by similar signalling pathways in human prostate cancer cells. Indeed, an elevated ARNT protein level was observed in hypoxic PC-3 cells. Interestingly, this effect was attenuated by inhibition of the phosphatidylinositol-3 kinase (PI3K)/AKT-pathway by Wortmannin [6]. Another hint regarding the ARNT expression pattern in cancer cells came from Skinner et al. [12]. Herein, the authors investigated the transcriptional regulation of VEGF in ovarian cancer cell lines in response to PI3K/Akt signalling. Blocking of this pathway using the compound LY294002 specifically inhibited HIF-1α expression but had no effect on ARNT. Unfortunately, the inducibility of ARNT in hypoxia was not tested in this study [12]. Most important, the observation that PI3K/Akt inhibition decreased HIF-1α but not ARNT in one model [12] whereas both transcription factors were reduced on protein level in another model [6] might suggest a HIF-dependent regulation of ARNT in certain cell lines.

The studies discussed so far clearly show that certain cell lines are capable to induce ARNT in hypoxia and that this effect is dependent on the experimental conditions (i.e. time points). Thus, one might assume that scientists became more aware of this phenomenon over time. However, ARNT was also used as a loading control in Western blot analysis [12, 13]. This application clearly demonstrates the major opinion of a complete non-hypoxic regulation of ARNT. Of note, effects of hypoxia and hypoxia mimetics on ARNT expression should be taken into consideration when studying the HIF pathway as previously proposed [1]. Such an approach will help to identify new cell types harbouring the hypoxia-inducible ARNT attribute and might provide novel mechanistic insights. The current proposed mechanism is discussed later in the chapter.

The seminal study conducted by Choi et al. shed light on ARNT expression and turnover [14]. The authors assumed that the regulation of ARNT expression or activity might significantly affect cell metabolism. Thus, ARNT should be regarded as a drug target and appropriate compounds need to be investigated. De novo synthesis of ARNT, enhanced stability of the protein and dimerisation with HIF-1α, represents three ways how this transcription factor can be controlled. Curcumin, the major component of the spice turmeric, was tested in this study for potential inhibitory effects on HIF-1. Interestingly, curcumin facilitated the degradation of ARNT and blocked HIF signalling [14]. Similar effects were reported by Ströfer et al. [15]. Curcumin-mediated ARNT depletion was observed in human HepG2, Hep3B and MCF-7 cells [15]. The half-life of ARNT was determined in Hep3B cells after cycloheximide treatment and calculated with approximately 5 h [14]. In contrast, curcumin exposure decreased ARNT half-life to roughly 2 h. It turned out that the curcumin-dependent degradation of ARNT was redox sensitive and could be reversed by antioxidants and the proteasome inhibitor MG-132 [14]. Remarkably, MG-132 did not affect ARNT protein level in the absence of curcumin. Therefore, the authors proposed the existence of two different mechanisms mediating ARNT turnover: a proteasome-independent mechanism under physiological conditions and a proteasome-dependent degradation in response to stress [14].

The elevation of ARNT protein expression under oxygen deprivation might not be an exclusive trait of cell lines. Exposure of primary mouse keratinocytes to acute hypoxia (1% O_2) resulted in an upregulation of ARNT after 4 and 5 h, respectively [16]. However, this effect was not statistically significant. Putative alterations on ARNT mRNA expression were also evaluated in this cell model. In contrast, time-course experiments revealed no apparent changes on mRNA level in murine keratinocytes cultured in hypoxia up to 48 h [16]. The selection of an inappropriate internal control in qPCR analysis can also lead to different expression levels in normoxia and hypoxia [17]. Therefore, Vavilala et al. determined the expression level of three housekeeping genes (ribosomal protein L32, β-actin and GAPDH) in normoxic and hypoxic cells, respectively [17]. The authors observed no significant changes on mRNA levels between both experimental settings. The aim of this study was to investigate inhibitory effects of Honokiol, a biphenolic phytochemical compound, on HIF signalling in several cell lines. The results presented in this report consist solely of gene expression data. Among them, the HIF-1α, HIF-2α and ARNT mRNA level were compared under normoxic and hypoxic conditions [17]. Remarkably, an approximately 7-fold increase in ARNT mRNA was observed in D407 human retinal pigment epithelial cells. In addition, a 2-fold upregulation was detected in HT-29 cells and a slight increase in the HEK293 cell line. MCF-7 cells showed no increase in ARNT mRNA due to hypoxic exposure. Unfortunately, the comparison of these effects among the cell lines tested in this study is limited because of different time points used (12 versus 24 h in D407 cells; 1% O_2) [17]. Nevertheless, the study provides clear evidence of a cell-specific transcriptional ARNT upregulation in hypoxia although these findings were not confirmed by Western blotting.

Further mechanistic insights into this cellular trait were provided by a research project investigating the regulation of ARNT in human melanoma cells [2]. Among a panel of five different cell lines, ARNT was rapidly elevated on protein level in 518A2 cells after treatment with the hypoxia mimetic cobalt chloride ($CoCl_2$). Interestingly, knockdown of HIF-1α in $CoCl_2$ stimulated and hypoxic 518A2 cells abolished the hypoxia-dependent upregulation of ARNT. Overexpression of a dominant-negative HIF mutant in this cell model indicated that ARNT expression is dependent on the HIF pathway itself. In agreement with these findings, overexpression of HIF-1α caused an elevation of ARNT protein in $CoCl_2$ treated 518A2 cells. Taken together, this study demonstrated a regulatory relationship between HIF-1α and its binding partner ARNT for the first time. In addition, it was concluded that this capability might prevent ARNT to become a limiting factor in hypoxia [2].

The first comprehensive study aiming to re-evaluate the regulation of ARNT was conducted by Wolff et al. [4]. Herein, numerous cell lines were exposed to 1 and 3% O_2 for different time points. In addition, hypoxia mimetics such as $CoCl_2$ and dimethyloxalylglycine (DMOG) were used and the quantity of ARNT protein determined by Western blotting. The authors found out that ARNT expression was induced in MCF-7, HeLa and Hep3B cells. Interestingly, the ARNT level was also dependent on the hypoxic environment used. A concentration of 1% O_2 led to a faster increase in ARNT protein but also to an earlier decline to basal levels as compared to 3% hypoxia. Moreover, the appropriate mRNA levels did not correlate with the amount of protein detected. In particular, in MCF-7 and Hep3B cells, a downregulation of ARNT mRNA was observed due to hypoxia. Therefore, the authors hypothesised the existence of a reciprocal feedback regulation between ARNT protein stability and de novo synthesis. This study provides convincing evidence that the predominant point of view that ARNT is unaffected by hypoxia and hypoxia mimetics cannot be applied to all cell lines in general [4].

The first review highlighting the topic of hypoxia-inducible ARNT was published by Mandl and Depping [1]. Herein, two major questions were raised: (1) How can cells acquire this attribute? and (2) What is the benefit for these cells? [1] Both issues will be discussed below. An updated list of cell lines capable to elevate ARNT in response to hypoxia is presented in **Table 1**. Among them, the human Hep3B cell line is obviously the best studied model in this context.

Cell line	Species	Origin	References
518A2	Human	Melanoma	[2]
A375	Human	Melanoma	[2]
D407*	Human	Retinal pigment epithelium	[17]
HEK-293*	Human	Embryonic kidney	[17]
HeLa	Human	Cervix adenocarcinoma	[4]
Hep3B	Human	Hepatoma	[3–5]
Hepa1	Mouse	Hepatoma	[7]
HT-29*	Human	Colorectal adenocarcinoma	[17]
L929	Mouse	Connective tissue	[7]
LNCaP*	Human	Prostate cancer	[20]
MCF-7	Human	Breast carcinoma	[4]
PC-3	Human	Prostate cancer	[20, 6]

*Only shown on mRNA level.

Table 1. Cell lines with hypoxia-inducible ARNT expression.

2.1.1. Purpose of hypoxia-inducible ARNT

The capability of certain tumour cells to upregulate ARNT under hypoxic conditions might provide a specific survival advantage as previously proposed [1]. Indeed, we recently discovered a relationship between ARNT and the cellular response to radiation [18]. Tumour hypoxia is associated with radioresistance and poor patient prognosis. Therefore, we investigated the effects of an altered expression of ARNT on radioresistance and performed clonogenic survival assays. As expected, silencing of ARNT in Hep3B and MCF-7 cells by siRNA rendered these models susceptible to radiation. Interestingly, overexpression of ARNT in these cell lines promoted radioresistance. Therefore, it was hypothesised that radiation treatment might provide a selection pressure and lead to an enrichment of high-ARNT expressing cells. Taken together, these findings provide evidence to consider ARNT as a drug target in order to increase radiosensitivity in tumour cells and as a predictive marker in this context [18].

As outlined above, there is evidence that HIF-1α mediates the elevation of ARNT under hypoxic conditions in certain cell lines. This regulatory relationship is the prerequisite of a feed-forward loop (FFL) as demonstrated recently in Hep3B cells. In such a network motif, one transcription factor regulates the other and both controls the expression of a target gene cooperatively. Given the fact that HIF-1α and ARNT form the transcriptional active complex HIF-1, which regulates a plethora of target genes, the FFL definition is fulfilled. By using reporter gene assays, we were able to demonstrate that overexpression of ARNT in Hep3B cells increased the luciferase signal in hypoxia. Therefore, it was concluded that augmented HIF signalling in terms of elevated target gene expression might be beneficial for tumour cells. These findings support the concept of ARNT being a limiting factor in at least certain cell models [3].

Moreover, general considerations regarding inducible gene expression are in line with the studies discussed above. In order to respond rapidly to micro-environmental alterations required genes need to be specifically activated. Inducible genes are highly regulated and must be quickly shut down to basal expression levels once the stimulus disappeared [19].

2.1.2. Mechanism of hypoxia-dependent ARNT upregulation

The mechanism(s) underlying this unique cellular attribute is (are) unclear. There is mounting evidence indicating a pivotal role of HIF-1α [2–4]. It was demonstrated that ARNT was increased in 518A2 human melanoma cells in a HIF-1α-dependent manner under hypoxic conditions [2]. A very similar mechanism was revealed in Hep3B cells [3]. Knockdown and overexpression of HIF-1α affected the ARNT protein level accordingly. Moreover, a clear transcriptional relationship between HIF-1α and its binding partner ARNT was established in this model system. Treatment with actinomycin D, an inhibitor of RNA synthesis, diminished the induction of ARNT under oxygen deprivation. In addition, appropriate gene-silencing experiments and qRT-PCR analysis confirmed this finding [3]. Another important observation might designate HIF-1α as a mediator of this cellular attribute. The PI3K/Akt inhibitor LY294002 was shown to inhibit HIF-1α expression in ovarian cancer cell lines but had no effect on ARNT protein [12]. In contrast, several independent studies have shown that the hypoxia-dependent increase in ARNT was abolished by blocking the PI3K/Akt pathway with LY294002 or similar compounds [2, 6, 20]. This finding—the susceptibility of ARNT to PI3K/Akt inhibition in certain models—might be characteristic for cells capable to induce ARNT in hypoxia. Taken together, this suggests a linear model and might imply ARNT to be a downstream target of HIF-1α.

The cellular cause of the regulatory relationship between HIF-1α and ARNT is not known. HIF-1α can act independent of its binding partner ARNT and regulate gene expression [1].

It was shown that HIF-1α can act as a co-activator or co-repressor on certain genes. In addition, an indirect regulatory connection between both transcription factors might exist [1]. HIF-regulated genes encode for growth factors, glucose transporters, glycolytic enzymes but also other transcription factors and miRNAs. Therefore, HIF-controlled transcription factors and miRNAs might influence ARNT expression [1, 3]. A general working concept is discussed below.

2.1.2.1. Working concept of hypoxia-inducible ARNT

Based on the studies mentioned above, a general working concept can be deduced (**Figure 1**). In addition to its oxygen regulation, the HIF pathway, that is, HIF-1α, is also controlled by growth factors via the PI3K/Akt signalling cascade leading to elevated translation [21, 22]. Upon activation HIF-1α induces the upregulation of its binding partner ARNT either on mRNA and/or protein level in appropriate cell lines. For instance, it was shown that hypoxic induction of ARNT in Hep3B cells is mediated by de novo synthesis [3]. This effect can be achieved either directly or indirectly. A direct mechanism might involve the recruitment of HIF-1α to the ARNT promoter, whereas an indirect mechanism might be mediated by other HIF-regulated transcription factors or miRNAs [1]. Indeed, a complex mutual regulatory relationship between miRNAs and PAS proteins exists. However, the physiological and pathophysiological mechanisms behind are unclear [23].

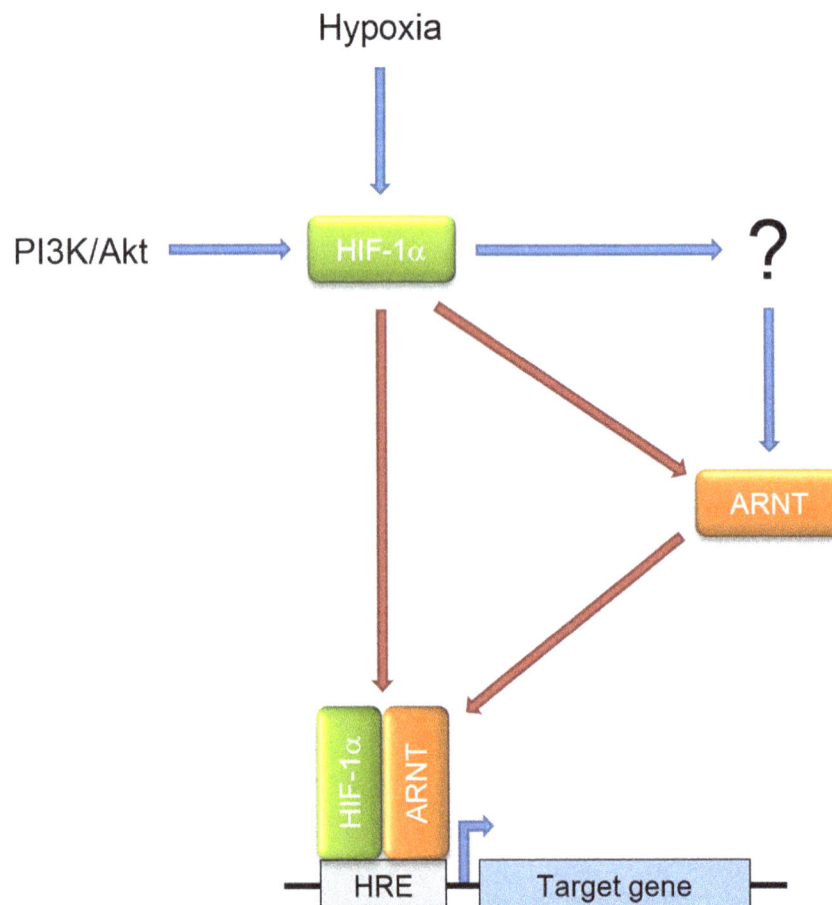

Figure 1. General working concept of hypoxia-inducible ARNT. See text for details.

Our recent experiments revealed that HIF-1α and ARNT are recruited to the ARNT gene promoter in hypoxic Hep3B cells. Deployment of CRISPR/Cas9 gene editing technology confirmed the importance of a unique genomic sequence for hypoxia-dependent ARNT upregulation. Therefore, these findings suggest a direct mechanism and render ARNT a putative HIF-1 target gene in Hep3B cells (unpublished observations; manuscript in preparation).

The regulatory relationship between HIF-1α and ARNT is part of a feed-forward loop (FFL; **Figure 1**: red arrows) as already demonstrated in Hep3B cells [3]. Subsequently, HIF-1α and its binding partner ARNT form the transcriptional active heterodimer HIF-1 and initiate the expression of various target genes. Therefore, an increased target gene expression seems to be beneficial for tumour cells [3].

2.1.3. Experimental conditions

Although the hypoxic inducibility of ARNT is described in specific cell lines by convincing data, not every study could confirm this circumstance. This obvious conflict depends mainly on the experimental conditions used. For instance, it was demonstrated that in Hep3B cells, 3% O_2 for 8 h was sufficient to elevate ARNT on protein level [3]. In contrast, a peak induction on mRNA level was observed after 5 h in the same setting [3]. Of note, these conditions need not to be appropriate in other cells. Until now, a few studies reported that ARNT mRNA and protein levels do not correlate in a number of cell lines [4, 18].

2.2. Regulation of ARNT by other factors

The regulation of ARNT or whether it responds to stimulation is poorly understood. There is evidence that ARNT expression is controlled by the NF-κB pathway in different models. It was demonstrated that ARNT mRNA was induced in HEK293 cells due to TNF-α stimulation. This effect was abrogated by pharmacological blocking or silencing of the NF-κB cascade [24]. Moreover, Per-ARNT-Sim (PAS) transcription factors belonging to different signalling circuits can compete for common binding partners such as ARNT (discussed below). Thus, misregulation of these proteins might contribute to tumour survival [9]. Noteworthily, the mutual regulation of PAS transcription factors on mRNA level was also mentioned in the literature, but appropriate citations are missing [22].

3. Crosstalk between Per-ARNT-Sim transcription factors

The HIF, AhR and BMAL1/Clock pathways respond to a decline in cellular oxygen concentration, environmental xenobiotics or govern circadian rhythms, respectively. All of these transcription factors are related. They belong to the group of Per-ARNT-Sim (PAS) transcription factors which are characterised by the presence of a PAS domain (composed of PAS-A and PAS-B subdomains) required for protein-protein interactions. Therefore, all family members are able to form homo- and heterodimers among the group [9, 25].

The transcription factor ARNT plays a pivotal role within the HIF and AhR pathways. It serves as the common binding partner for HIF-α subunits and ligands activated AhR proteins [1].

Therefore, a competition between both signalling cascades regarding the recruitment of ARNT might be obvious. Indeed, early evidence for such an antagonism was provided by Gradin et al. [26]. By using luciferase reporter gene constructs under the control of xenobi-otic-responsive elements (XRE), the effect of HIF and AhR activation was studied in HepG2 cells. As expected, stimulation of cells with an appropriate AhR ligand leads to a pronounced induction of reporter gene expression. This effect was suppressed by co-treatment with the hypoxia mimetic cobalt chloride. Co-immunoprecipitation experiments clearly indicated a competition between the HIF and AhR pathway relating to ARNT binding. In addition, it was shown that HIF-1α could efficiently compete with the AhR for dimerisation with ARNT. This study provided evidence for a HIF-1α-mediated inhibition of AhR signalling by sequestra-tion of ARNT [26]. Vorrink et al. [27] observed similar effects again in human hepatocellular carcinoma HepG2 cells and in the human keratinocyte HaCaT cell line. One major advantage of this study was the genuine hypoxic exposure of cells instead of stimulation with hypoxia mimetics such as cobalt chloride. AhR signalling was triggered by treatment with the dioxin-like compound PCB126. Again, hypoxia inhibited CYP1A1 reporter gene activity in PCB126 stimulated HepG2 cells. Importantly, ARNT overexpression caused an elevated luminescence signal under normoxic and hypoxic conditions. Moreover, forced ARNT expression was suf-ficient to overcome the inhibitory effect of hypoxia on AhR signalling. The authors concluded that ARNT is sequestered by HIF-1α in hypoxia thus limiting the availability of this transcrip-tion factor for AhR heterodimerisation [27]. Noteworthily, another report published nearly two decades ago claims the complete opposite [28]. This study might provide evidence for a lack of competition between HIF and AhR signalling on ARNT recruitment. Unfortunately, the presented arguments and data are not convincing at many points [28].

Furthermore, a crosstalk between AhR and BMAL1/Clock exists. Lipophilic AhR ligands such as dioxin or dietary polyphenols bind within the AhR PAS-B domain and trigger nuclear trans-location. Within the nucleus activated AhR can dimerise with BMAL1 thus disrupting the auto-regulatory loop of BMAL1/Clock genes. Therefore, AhR activation leads to a suppression of circadian rhythms, whereas AhR inhibition strengthens rhythm amplitude [25]. Interestingly, there is evidence that both AhR and ARNT are expressed in an oscillatory pattern in vivo [29].

4. Subcellular dynamics of ARNT and turnover

Translocation of ARNT from the cytoplasm into the nucleus is mediated by importins as also demonstrated for other HIF family members [30, 31]. Blocking of this specific process was proposed as a novel way to suppress HIF signalling [30]. Whether ARNT shuttles, back into the cytoplasm is unknown. Under these circumstances, inhibition of the putative nuclear export might prolong HIF activity. Moreover, whether ARNT is degraded, within the nucleus is not investigated in greater depth (depicted in **Figure 2**).

In general, there is evidence for two different mechanisms leading to ARNT degradation. It was found out that ARNT was not affected by the proteasome inhibitor MG-132 under physiological conditions. In contrast, proteasomal degradation of ARNT might be triggered by reactive oxygen species [3, 14].

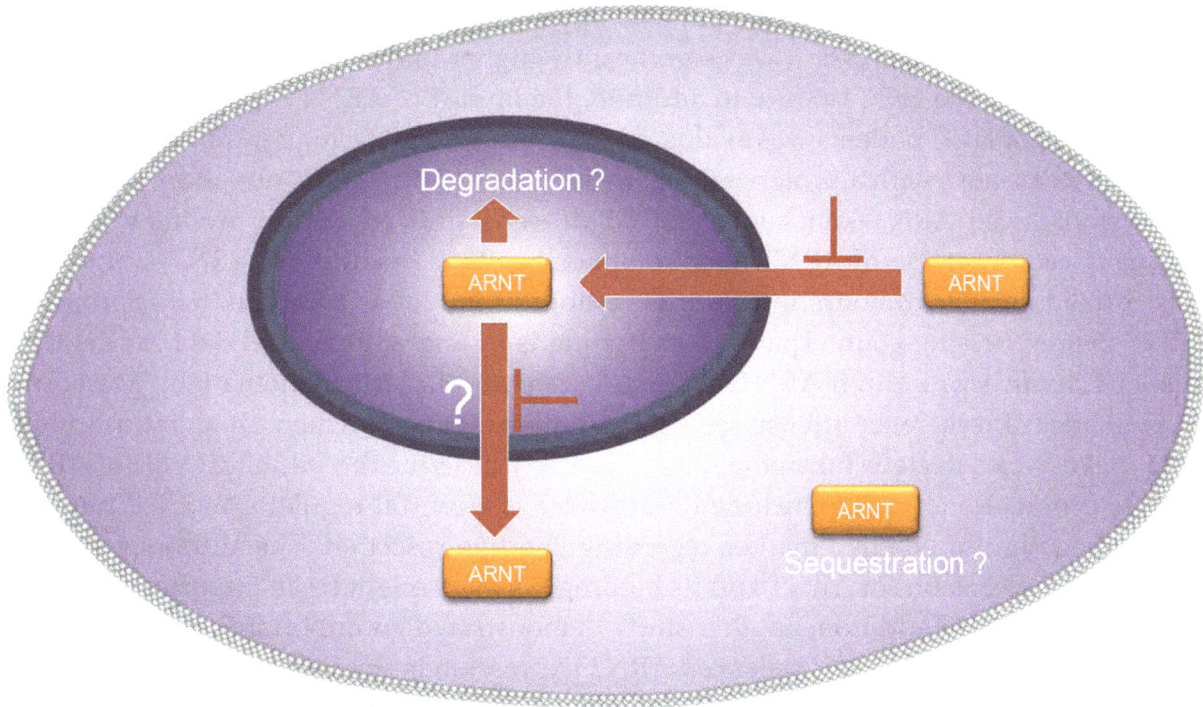

Figure 2. Subcellular logistics of ARNT. See text for details.

5. Clinical aspects

Inhibition of the HIF pathway is proposed as a treatment strategy in oncology. Several appropriate compounds have been identified and confirmed in xenograft models. These drugs are able to block different processes of the HIF signalling pathway. For instance, HIF-1α protein synthesis is diminished by rapamycin which is an inhibitor of mTOR. The antibiotic acriflavine prevents heterodimerisation of HIF-1α and ARNT subunits [32]. Moreover, a plethora of other HIF inhibitors was discovered which comprise of different chemical entities. HIF is considered as an attractive drug target, and blocking of its activity might lead to cytostatic antitumour effects. A synergistic outcome with radiotherapy is also expected [33, 34]. However, such drugs might be useful in multidrug regimes only in a subset of cancer patients. Cancers in which HIF is a strong driving force for disease progression are assumed to be susceptible for anti-HIF treatment [32].

The temporal importance of ARNT during tumour growth was investigated by Shi et al. [35]. Herein, the authors used murine hepatoma Hepa-1 cells transduced with a Tet-Off mArnt construct. Xenograft experiments conducted with these cells indicated that ARNT is particularly required during the early stage of tumour growth. The authors proposed that a profound inhibition of the HIF pathway might be achieved only by suppressing both HIF-1α and HIF-2α proteins. Therefore, it was concluded that the binding partner ARNT might represent a preferable therapeutic target rather than HIF-α subunits [35]. More convincing evidence regarding the role of ARNT in this malignancy was provided by a study using human tissue samples and cell lines [36]. ARNT expression was analysed by immunohistochemistry in hepatocellular carcinoma (HCC) and liver tissues. ARNT was found primarily in the nucleus but also in the cytoplasm in a minor fraction of cells. Interestingly, ARNT expression was significantly higher in normal liver samples as compared to appropriate HCC tissues. In addition, the impact of ARNT expression on overall survival (OS) of HCC patients was evaluated [36]. Surprisingly, a high intra-tumour ARNT level was associated with a prolonged OS. In agreement with this observation, stably lentiviral transduced ARNT-knockdown HCCLM6 cells showed a high proliferation rate, whereas overexpression of ARNT had the opposite effect. In addition, ARNT-suppressed cells formed smaller tumours in a murine xenograft model as compared to appropriate ARNT-overexpressing counterparts. This finding is in line with clinical data indicating a smaller tumour size in high-ARNT expressing hepatocellular carcinoma [36]. Moreover, the incidence of recurrence after surgery was significantly lower when a high intra-tumour ARNT level was detected. Taken together, this study describes an inhibitory role of ARNT in HCC progression. It was concluded that ARNT is a central regulator in HCC progression and a useful predictive marker regarding curative resection. The authors proposed that the relative balance of ARNT and its binding partners might be an important determinant in HCC [36]. In addition, another study demonstrated an important role of ARNT in this malignancy. Choi et al. [37] silenced ARNT expression in several human hepatoma cell lines by using siRNA and evaluated the effects on cell growth. It was shown that knockdown of this transcription factor inhibited proliferation and sensitised cells to apoptosis [37]. An elegant approach to target ARNT by small molecule inhibitors was conducted by Guo et al. [38]. Herein, nuclear magnetic resonance and biochemical screens were used in order to identify molecules selectively binding to the PAS domain of ARNT. The compound KG-548 was discovered to compete with the co-activator TACC3 for ARNT binding. The specific blocking of protein-protein interactions among transcription factors represents a novel technique to inhibit HIF signalling. Due to the shared use of ARNT among alpha subunits, targeting this protein was proposed to be more efficient as compared to its counterparts [38]. Evidence highlighting the importance of ARNT as a drug target was also provided by another study. Chan and colleagues [39] described that ARNT expression enhances cisplatin resistance in cancer cells. This phenotype was mediated by upregulation of MDR1, a multidrug efflux pump of the ABC superfamily, by a direct mechanism. Accordingly, knockdown of ARNT by siRNA transfection reduced cisplatin resistance in human cancer cells. Moreover, ARNT silencing increased the therapeutic efficacy of this cytotoxic drug in a murine xenograft model [39].

Targeting the HIF pathway in cancer therapy in order to achieve tumour control has been proposed by several reports [40–42]. Remarkably, the majority of HIF inhibitors described until now lack specificity. For instance, the drug topotecan blocks topoisomerase I activity but also diminished HIF signalling in preclinical models. This inhibitory effect on HIF was accomplished by preventing the accumulation of HIF-1α. In multihistology target-driven clinical trial, Kummar et al. [43] evaluated the oral use of this compound in a small number of cancer patients. Different tumour entities were diagnosed in these patients including ovarian cancer, sarcoma and melanoma among others. A complete inhibition of HIF-1α was detected in biopsies of a few patients, but inherent sampling and heterogeneous HIF-1α expression might limit this finding [43]. In contrast, despite the clear role of ARNT in tumour progression, its drug-ability and appropriate treatment effects need to be evaluated in a clinical setting.

6. Concluding remarks

The attribute of certain tumour cells to elevate the transcription factor ARNT in hypoxia was shown decades ago but since neglected in HIF biology. Only a small number of studies focus on the regulation of ARNT, especially under hypoxic conditions. Therefore, hypoxia-inducible ARNT is an emerging concept in this field. According to the major opinion, ARNT is a constitutively expressed gene. This means that ARNT expression is not effected by environmental factors such as hypoxia. Due to the fact that there are exceptions from this dogma, the statement of a constitutive ARNT expression should be revised and not used in general terms. Thus, ARNT should be regarded as a "cell-specific facultative gene" in tumour cells which indicates an expression as needed.

Author details

Markus Mandl and Reinhard Depping*

*Address all correspondence to: reinhard.depping@uni-luebeck.de

Institute of Physiology, Center for Structural and Cell Biology in Medicine, University of Luebeck, Luebeck, Germany

References

[1] Mandl M, Depping R. (2014). Hypoxia-inducible aryl hydrocarbon receptor nuclear translocator (ARNT) (HIF-1beta): is it a rare exception? *Molecular Medicine (Cambridge, Mass)* 20: 215–220.

[2] Mandl M, Kapeller B, Lieber R, Macfelda K. (2013). Hypoxia-inducible factor-1beta (HIF-1beta) is upregulated in a HIF-1alpha-dependent manner in 518A2 human melanoma cells under hypoxic conditions. *Biochemical and Biophysical Research Communications* 434: 166–172.

[3] Mandl M, Lieberum MK, Depping R. (2016). A HIF-1alpha-driven feed-forward loop augments HIF signalling in Hep3B cells by upregulation of ARNT. *Cell Death & Disease* 7: e2284.

[4] Wolff M, Jelkmann W, Dunst J, Depping R. (2013). The aryl hydrocarbon receptor nuclear translocator (ARNT/HIF-1beta) is influenced by hypoxia and hypoxia-mimetics. *Cellular Physiology and Biochemistry* 32: 849–858.

[5] Wang GL, Jiang BH, Rue EA, Semenza GL. (1995). Hypoxia-inducible factor 1 is a basic-helix-loop-helix-PAS heterodimer regulated by cellular O_2 tension. *Proceedings of the National Academy of Sciences of the United States of America* 92: 5510–5514.

[6] Zhong H, Hanrahan C, van der Poel H, Simons JW. (2001). Hypoxia-inducible factor 1alpha and 1beta proteins share common signaling pathways in human prostate cancer cells. *Biochemical and Biophysical Research Communications* 284: 352–356.

[7] Chilov D, Camenisch G, Kvietikova I, Ziegler U, Gassmann M, Wenger RH. (1999). Induction and nuclear translocation of hypoxia-inducible factor-1 (HIF-1): heterodimerization with ARNT is not necessary for nuclear accumulation of HIF-1alpha. *Journal of Cell Science* 112(Pt 8): 1203–1212.

[8] Kimura Y, Kasamatsu A, Nakashima D, et al. (2016). ARNT2 regulates tumoral growth in oral squamous cell carcinoma. *Journal of Cancer* 7: 702–710.

[9] Bersten DC, Sullivan AE, Peet DJ, Whitelaw ML. (2013). bHLH-PAS proteins in cancer. *Nature Reviews Cancer* 13: 827–841.

[10] Huang LE, Arany Z, Livingston DM, Bunn HF. (1996). Activation of hypoxia-inducible transcription factor depends primarily upon redox-sensitive stabilization of its alpha subunit. *The Journal of Biological Chemistry* 271: 32253–32259.

[11] Pientka FK, Hu J, Schindler SG, et al. (2012). Oxygen sensing by the prolyl-4-hydroxylase PHD2 within the nuclear compartment and the influence of compartmentalisation on HIF-1 signalling. *Journal of Cell Science* 125: 5168–5176.

[12] Skinner HD, Zheng JZ, Fang J, Agani F, Jiang BH. (2004). Vascular endothelial growth factor transcriptional activation is mediated by hypoxia-inducible factor 1alpha, HDM2, and p70S6K1 in response to phosphatidylinositol 3-kinase/AKT signaling. *The Journal of Biological Chemistry* 279: 45643–45651.

[13] Hu CJ, Wang LY, Chodosh LA, Keith B, Simon MC. (2003). Differential roles of hypoxia-inducible factor 1alpha (HIF-1alpha) and HIF-2alpha in hypoxic gene regulation. *Molecular and Cellular Biology* 23: 9361–9374.

[14] Choi H, Chun YS, Kim SW, Kim MS, Park JW. (2006). Curcumin inhibits hypoxia-inducible factor-1 by degrading aryl hydrocarbon receptor nuclear translocator: a mechanism of tumor growth inhibition. *Molecular Pharmacology* 70: 1664–1671.

[15] Strofer M, Jelkmann W, Depping R. (2011). Curcumin decreases survival of Hep3B liver and MCF-7 breast cancer cells: the role of HIF. *Strahlentherapie und Onkologie* 187: 393–400.

[16] Weir L, Robertson D, Leigh IM, Vass JK, Panteleyev AA. (2011). Hypoxia-mediated control of HIF/ARNT machinery in epidermal keratinocytes. *Biochimica et Biophysica Acta* 1813: 60–72.

[17] Vavilala DT, Ponnaluri VK, Vadlapatla RK, Pal D, Mitra AK, Mukherji M. (2012). Honokiol inhibits HIF pathway and hypoxia-induced expression of histone lysine demethylases. *Biochemical and Biophysical Research Communications* 422: 369–374.

[18] Mandl M, Lieberum MK, Dunst J, Depping R. (2015). The expression level of the transcription factor Aryl hydrocarbon receptor nuclear translocator (ARNT) determines cellular survival after radiation treatment. *Radiation Oncology (London, England)* 10: 229.

[19] Weake VM, Workman JL. (2010). Inducible gene expression: diverse regulatory mechanisms. *Nature Reviews Genetics* 11: 426–437.

[20] Huang S, Guo Y, Jacobi A, et al. (2016). Aromatic hydrocarbon receptor suppresses prostate cancer bone metastasis cells-induced vasculogenesis of endothelial progenitor cells under hypoxia. Cellular *Physiology and Biochemistry* 39: 709–720.

[21] Semenza GL. (2010). Oxygen homeostasis. *Wiley Interdisciplinary Reviews* 2: 336–361.

[22] Masoud GN, Li W. (2015). HIF-1alpha pathway: role, regulation and intervention for cancer therapy. *Acta Pharmaceutica Sinica* 5: 378–389.

[23] Li Y, Wei Y, Guo J, Cheng Y, He W. (2015). Interactional role of microRNAs and bHLH-PAS proteins in cancer (Review). *International Journal of Oncology* 47: 25–34.

[24] van Uden P, Kenneth NS, Webster R, Muller HA, Mudie S, Rocha S. (2011). Evolutionary conserved regulation of HIF-1beta by NF-kappaB. *PLoS Genetics* 7: e1001285.

[25] Jaeger C, Tischkau SA. (2016). Role of aryl hydrocarbon receptor in circadian clock disruption and metabolic dysfunction. *Environmental Health Insights* 10: 133–141.

[26] Gradin K, McGuire J, Wenger RH, et al. (1996). Functional interference between hypoxia and dioxin signal transduction pathways: competition for recruitment of the Arnt transcription factor. *Molecular and Cellular Biology* 16: 5221–5231.

[27] Vorrink SU, Severson PL, Kulak MV, Futscher BW, Domann FE. (2014). Hypoxia perturbs aryl hydrocarbon receptor signaling and CYP1A1 expression induced by PCB 126 in human skin and liver-derived cell lines. *Toxicology and Applied Pharmacology* 274: 408–416.

[28] Pollenz RS, Davarinos NA, Shearer TP. (1999). Analysis of aryl hydrocarbon receptor-mediated signaling during physiological hypoxia reveals lack of competition for the aryl hydrocarbon nuclear translocator transcription factor. *Molecular Pharmacology* 56: 1127–1137.

[29] Richardson VM, Santostefano MJ, Birnbaum LS. (1998). Daily cycle of bHLH-PAS proteins, Ah receptor and Arnt, in multiple tissues of female Sprague-Dawley rats. *Biochemical and Biophysical Research Communications* 252: 225–231.

[30] Depping R, Jelkmann W, Kosyna FK. (2015). Nuclear-cytoplasmatic shuttling of proteins in control of cellular oxygen sensing. *Journal of Molecular Medicine* 93: 599–608.

[31] Depping R, Steinhoff A, Schindler SG, et al. (2008). Nuclear translocation of hypoxia-inducible factors (HIFs): involvement of the classical importin alpha/beta pathway. *Biochimica et Biophysica Acta* 1783: 394–404.

[32] Semenza GL. (2012). Hypoxia-inducible factors in physiology and medicine. *Cell* 148: 399–408.

[33] Ban HS, Uto Y, Nakamura H. (2011). Hypoxia-inducible factor inhibitors: a survey of recent patented compounds (2004–2010). *Expert Opinion on Therapeutic Patents* 21: 131–146.

[34] Strofer M, Jelkmann W, Metzen E, Brockmeier U, Dunst J, Depping R. (2011). Stabilisation and knockdown of HIF--two distinct ways comparably important in radiotherapy. *Cellular Physiology and Biochemistry* 28: 805–812.

[35] Shi S, Yoon DY, Hodge-Bell K, Huerta-Yepez S, Hankinson O. (2010). Aryl hydrocarbon nuclear translocator (hypoxia inducible factor 1beta) activity is required more during early than late tumor growth. *Molecular Carcinogenesis* 49: 157–165.

[36] Liang Y, Li WW, Yang BW, et al. (2011). Aryl hydrocarbon receptor nuclear translocator is associated with tumor growth and progression of hepatocellular carcinoma. *International Journal of Cancer* 130: 1745–1754.

[37] Choi SH, Chung AR, Kang W, et al. (2014). Silencing of hypoxia-inducible factor-1beta induces anti-tumor effects in hepatoma cell lines under tumor hypoxia. *PLoS One* 9: e103304.

[38] Guo Y, Partch CL, Key J, et al. (2013). Regulating the ARNT/TACC3 axis: multiple approaches to manipulating protein/protein interactions with small molecules. *ACS Chemical Biology* 8: 626–635.

[39] Chan YY, Kalpana S, Chang WC, Chang WC, Chen BK. (2013). Expression of aryl hydrocarbon receptor nuclear translocator enhances cisplatin resistance by upregulating MDR1 expression in cancer cells. *Molecular Pharmacology* 84: 591–602.

[40] Milani M, Harris AL. (2008). Targeting tumour hypoxia in breast cancer. *European Journal of Cancer* 44: 2766–2773.

[41] Kizaka-Kondoh S, Tanaka S, Harada H, Hiraoka M. (2009). The HIF-1-active microenvironment: an environmental target for cancer therapy. *Advanced Drug Delivery Reviews* 61: 623–632.

[42] Wilson WR, Hay MP. (2011). Targeting hypoxia in cancer therapy. *Nature Reviews Cancer* 11: 393–410.

[43] Kummar S, Raffeld M, Juwara L, et al. (2011). Multihistology, target-driven pilot trial of oral topotecan as an inhibitor of hypoxia-inducible factor-1alpha in advanced solid tumors. *Clinical Cancer Research* 17: 5123–5131.

8

Role of the Hypoxia-Inducible Factor in Periodontal Inflammation

Xiao Xiao Wang, Yu Chen and Wai Keung Leung

Abstract

Human periodontitis is a chronic inflammatory disease induced by opportunistic Gram-negative anaerobic bacteria at the tooth-supporting apparatus. Within the gingivitis-affected sulcus or periodontal pocket, the resident anaerobic bacteria interact with the host inflammatory reactions leading to a lower oxygen or hypoxic environment. A cellular/tissue oxygen-sensing mechanism and its appropriate regulation are needed to assist tissue adaptation to natural/pathology-induced variations in oxygen availability. In this chapter, we reviewed the biological relevance of hypoxia in periodontal/oral cellular development, epithelial barrier function, periodontal inflammation, and immunity. The role of hypoxia-inducible factor-1α in pathogen-host cross talk and alveolar bone homeostasis was also discussed. The naturally occurring pathophysiological process of hypoxia appeared to entail fundamental relevance for periodontal defense and regeneration.

Keywords: cell hypoxia, chronic periodontitis, hypoxia-inducible factor-1, alpha subunit

1. Introduction

Regardless of the oxygen sources, when an animal acquires oxygen through its breathing apparatus, the oxygen will have to pass under a reducing partial oxygen pressure (pO_2) gradient from the source via circulation to different organs and then tissues and cells. In mammals, such as rats, inspired pO_2 is around 21.3 kPa at sea level. When blood flows through the alveolar capillaries, it drops to approximately 14 kPa and is then progressively reduced to 2.1, 1.3, and 0.27–3.3 kPa in the spleen, thymus, and retina, respectively [1, 2], while in the brain, it may be as low as 0.05–1.07 kPa, depending on the cranial location [3].

Due to the colonization by subgingival biofilm, oxygen is persistently consumed to various extents by the facultative anaerobic microbes within the periodontal sulcus (2.33–8.40 kPa). In the gingivitis-affected sulcus or periodontal pocket, the inflammation induced by the residential anaerobic bacteria with or without microulcerations or wounding leads to an even lower oxygen tension [4]. At the tissue level, the availability of oxygen is dependent on the distance from the oxygen-supplying blood vessels. Although the diffusion distance of oxygen *in vivo* is estimated to be 100–200 μm, a pO_2 of almost zero has been recorded in tissues 100 μm away from the nourishing blood vessels [5]. Therefore, a cellular/tissue oxygen-sensing mechanism is needed to assist tissue adaptation to nature/pathology-induced variations in oxygen availability.

In humans, a drop in oxygen concentration in the atmosphere is sensed by the carotid body at the bifurcation of the carotid arteries, which then increases the rate and depth of breathing. At the levels of tissues and cells, including the human periodontium, such adaptive responses to low oxygen tension or hypoxia are mainly mediated through a key cellular transcription factor named the hypoxia-inducible factor (HIF) [6].

2. Hypoxia in the oral/periodontal environment

Oxygen is an essential molecule for survival. Mammals—including humans—depend on oxygen for electron transport, oxidative phosphorylation, and energy generation. Variations in tissue oxygen needs are attributed to a number of physiological or pathological states, meaning that the tissues concerned have to be able to adapt to various O_2 environments including hypoxia. To survive, mammalian cells evolved in such a way that cellular O_2 availability or homeostasis could be monitored and tightly regulated [7]. This is made possible by a cellular HIF system. Cellular hypoxia, or a lower than "normal" concentration of O_2 in cells, occurs commonly and could induce significant changes, immediate or delayed, on cellular processes, including cell growth and apoptosis, cell proliferation and survival, pH regulation and energy metabolism, cell migration, matrix and barrier function, angiogenesis, and vasomotor regulation [8–13]. These biological processes involve active responses by the body to secure an additional oxygen supply via circulation. Such dynamic processes of cellular/tissue oxygen monitoring, O_2 consumption, and delivery, corresponding to the respective cellular/tissue functional state, are tightly controlled to ensure proper survival of the multicellular organism concerned [14].

As described earlier, the normal tissue/cellular pO_2 levels in mammals are dependent on their location and physiology and, hence, vary among different human body compartments and cell/tissue conditions [15]. Hypoxia in oral cells/tissues is, in fact, a common occurrence [6]. The local hypoxic microenvironment is considered a consequence of growth/development, wound healing, smoking habits, or concurrent oral inflammation/infection/diseases.

Taking oral cellular development/regeneration as an example, the blood vessel network is promoted by vascular endothelial growth factors (VEGF) secreted by stem cells from apical papilla under hypoxia, suggesting a role of hypoxia in pulp revascularization and bioengineered pulp replacements [16]. On the other hand, it is reported that extreme hypoxia-like response induced by the chemical cobalt chloride ($CoCl_2$) could stimulate periodontal ligament (PDL) stem cell cytotoxicity through mitochondria-apoptotic and autophagic pathways involving HIF-1α [17]. During pathological processes, it is reported that a low oxygen level may regulate cell migration of oral cancer cells, thus influencing the invasion and metastasis in malignant oral lesions [18].

With reference to growth, increasing evidence shows that certain hormonal regulation could be interfered with hypoxia or HIF [19]. For instance, it is reported that growth hormone expression in lymphocytes and parathyroid hormone-related protein in articular chondrocytes can be induced by hypoxia [20, 21]. We postulate that if similar biology could be expressed in the head and neck region, HIF or hypoxia may bring profound effects on the growth and development of orofacial structures.

3. Hypoxia and chronic periodontal inflammation

Metabolic shifts under hypoxia are common occurrences in the periodontal inflammatory process as a result of the imbalance between the tissue oxygen supply and consumption [22]. The accumulation of intracellular HIF-1 promotes the transcription of a spectrum of genes to maintain cellular homeostasis. Hypoxia induces the expression of a number of angiogenic factors to improve the blood supply in needed areas including inflamed periodontium [6]. These include VEGF, platelet-derived growth factor (PDGF), and angioprotein-1 and -2. Related genes produce controlling perfusion, such as the PDGF-β receptor, cyclooxygenase-2, and nitric oxide synthase (NOS), of which NOS modulates vascular smooth muscle cells' functions and reacts to changes in the cellular HIF-1 level [23]. Moreover, HIF activation promotes a metabolic switch to reduce oxygen consumption by shifting energy metabolism from aerobic respiration to glycolysis. Activation of HIF also upregulates the expression of pyruvate dehydrogenase kinase, which reduces the incorporation of pyruvate into the citric acid cycle [24]. This metabolic switch is essential for the hosts' defense because such HIF-1α–regulated glycolytic metabolism is required in B cell development [25] and T cell metabolism [26].

Under a chronic inflammatory state, hypoxia induces protective cellular responses or a local defense. However, if the cause of inflammation cannot be eradicated, such hypoxic cell/tissue reactions contribute to the pathophysiology of inflammation and, hence, disease pathogenesis [27]. A similar scenario can be observed within the human periodontium in periodontitis. Periodontitis is characterized by chronic inflammation of the tooth-supporting tissues, initiated by a multitude of Gram-negative anaerobic pathogens including *Aggregatibacter actinomycetemcomitans*, *Porphyromonas gingivalis*, *Tannerella forsythia*, *Treponema denticola*, and so on [28]. At sites where a chronic inflammatory reaction could be found, oxygen consumption is elevated and blood perfusion is stimulated, but the actual local microcirculation could be compromised [29]. This local tissue pO_2 change is partly due to increased oxygen consumption, including oxygen usage by both resident cells and infiltrated defense cells, and partly because of diminished oxygen availability due to endothelial damage and vasoconstricted microcirculation.

Local hypoxia in periodontitis in turn enhances the anaerobic Gram-negative pathogens' survival and further lowers the oxygen tension at the vicinity. The tissue hypoxia in periodontal disease has been characterized by increased HIF-1α protein that is detectable in periodontitis-affected tissue biopsies using Western blot and anti–HIF-1α immunostaining [6, 30]. Myeloid cell lineage of HIF-1$\alpha^{-/-}$ (deprived) mice had impaired immune effector molecules, such as nitric oxide (NO) and tumor necrosis factor-alpha (TNF-α) production, thus reducing their bactericidal capability [31]. Therefore, the ability to adapt to a reduced oxygen supply, which maintains immune cell surveillance capability in all tissue environments, is important and necessary in the successful elimination of pathogens [32].

Proinflammatory cytokines and matrix metalloproteinases (MMPs) act as mediators for the inflammation process or play a role in extracellular matrix degradation, respectively. Researchers often investigate the levels of such biological markers in the periodontium in attempts to gauge the severity of periodontal disease and monitor periodontal treatment outcomes [33]. Recent studies reported that a hypoxic environment may upregulate proinflammatory cytokines and MMPs' expression from host cells during periodontal disease [34]. The idea was that hypoxia further encourages lipopolysaccharide (LPS)-induced TNF-α, interleukin-1β, and interleukin 6 (IL-6) expressions via LPS toll-like receptor (TLR) interaction that, in turn, activates the nuclear factor kappa B (NF-κB) pathway in human PDL cells upon exposure to the aforementioned Gram-negative bacterial surface component [35–37].

At the collagen destruction front, periodontal epithelial cells could produce MMPs in response to bacteria-induced activation of pathogen-associated molecular patterns (PAMP) including TLRs. These host enzymes contribute to the extracellular matrix degradation that accommodates local inflammatory reactions, as well as the later tissue remodeling that ensues once inflammation stops [38, 39]. Inhibition of HIF-1α activity by chetomin, a *Chaetomium* metabolite that can incapacitate tumor cells' hypoxic adaptation or knockdown HIF-1α gene expression by small, interfering RNA, could markedly attenuate the production of LPS- and nicotine-stimulated MMPs and prostaglandin E$_2$ from PDL cells. Such observations suggest the possibility of HIF-1α being a potential target in periodontal tissue destruction associated with smoking and dental plaque [40]. Further supporting the idea that hypoxia may be one of the key biological responses in periodontal inflammation.

Certain periodontopathogens, other than acting as effective mediators of periodontal inflammation, are capable of doing more harm to a host under a low pO$_2$ environment. For instance, *P. gingivalis* LPS under hypoxia increases PDL fibroblasts' oxidative stress and induces a reduction of catalase, indicating a collapse of the protective machinery favoring the increase in reactive oxygen species (ROS) and the progression of inflammatory oral diseases [41].

Considering the healing of oral wounds, several studies reported that the biological process in general could be enhanced or accelerated under hypoxia via HIF-1 [42, 43]. For example, the wound healing of rat palatal mucosa was enhanced by the hydroxylase inhibitor dimethyloxalylglycine, a HIF-1α stabilizer, under a hypoxic environment, and this enzyme was reported to induce hypoxia-mimetic angiogenesis [44]. With reference to hard tissue healing, $CoCl_2$ triggered the expression of angiogenic mediators and bone turnover-related genes, which promoted fracture healing and repair *in vivo* [45]. The research report also indicated that, during distraction osteogenesis, an angiogenic effect and bone healing could be promoted by conditioned media collected from dental pulp cells under hypoxia [46]. These findings implied the possibility that a low tissue oxygen level may act as a biological signal, promoting soft and hard tissue healing, including that of the orofacial regions, mediated through inflammation.

4. Hypoxia and periodontal immunity

Hypoxic responses or HIF is reported to be strongly related to innate human responses, with low oxygen modulating energy metabolism and various genes' expression within defense cells that, in turn, dictate the immune performance and the host protection outcomes [47]. The biological impact of low pO_2 on T cells' functions was reflected by the HIF-1– and adenosine receptor–modulated effects [48]. Indeed, both lymphocytes and myeloid cells were affected and the hypoxia-induced adaptive immune response changes would interfere or affect the innate immunity. The relevance of hypoxia in pathological processes was well established upon the appreciation that wounds, infectious loci, and tumor growth each involved extremely low oxygen tension [1].

It has been well appreciated that low oxygen tension is common at inflamed periodontitis sites [4]; thus, the corresponding local immune responses must adapt to the hypoxic challenges. As mentioned above, hypoxia plays an important role in modulating the cellular activities of innate and adaptive immunity, so the impact of low pO_2 in periodontal immune responses is quite significant.

Oral innate immunity is the first line of defense against periodontopathogens, which functions to recognize, attenuate, and eliminate the nonself invaders and to trigger downstream immune responses. Granulocytes and monocytes/macrophages are the main cell types for innate periodontal immunity [49, 50]. When extensive inflammation takes place, these cells have to travel into the tissue compartment with low pO_2 (i.e., the infected area) to provide defense and wall-off the invasion. To prevent the invasion, intense energy metabolism has to occur within the involved innate defense cells. An appropriate hypoxic cellular reaction and adaptation is, therefore, very important in the periodontal innate immune cells, which develop functional and survival responses regulated by the oxygen sensor HIF [51].

Defense cells rely heavily on glycolysis for the production of ATP to compensate for the limited oxidative metabolism in hypoxia. Immune cell energy metabolism appeared to significantly influence its corresponding response. As a critical modulator for the expression of glycolytic enzymes, the absence of HIF-1α leads to a significant reduction of ATP availability in myeloid cells [52]. It was reported that a knockdown of HIF-1α protein led to a nullified IL-6 production when exposed to LPS, suggesting that HIF-1α supported the LPS-dependent expression of IL-6 that, in turn, prevented the depletion of ATP and, therefore, protected myeloid cells against LPS/TLR4-induced apoptosis [53]. In human monocytes, LPS and hypoxia synergistically activated HIF-1 through p44/42 mitogen-activated protein kinases (MAPK) and NF-κB; however, repetitive exposure to LPS could induce tolerance to bacterial endotoxins and, hence, impair corresponding HIF-1α induction, which reduces the ability of monocytic cells to survive and function under low oxygen [54, 55].

To combat invading pathogens, HIF also promotes polymorphonuclear neutrophil (PMN) recruitment via the restoration of blood flow at inflamed tissues and enhances neovascularization. With hypoxia, the HIF restored perfusion also facilitates PMNs' diapedesis [56, 57]. Furthermore, PMN apoptosis was attenuated under hypoxia, with HIF-1α reported to be a protective factor in the regulation of its functional longevity [58]. Such longevity regulation involved NF-κB signaling that was found to be essential in constitutive HIF-1 protein translation [58, 59].

The cellular stress-related transcription factor NF-κB is closely related to hypoxia despite the fact that the relationship is not yet completely understood. It was reported that classical or canonical NF-κB activation under the stress of hypoxia often involves the activation of transforming growth factor-B-activating kinase and the inhibitor of κB kinase (IKK) complex [60]. In addition to classical NF-κB signaling, the noncanonical NF-κB pathway could be activated by hypoxia independent of HIF-1α via NF-κB-inducing kinase and IKK homodimer activation [61]. ROS, a key inflammatory regulator in chronic periodontal inflammation, is confirmed to mediate HIF-1α induction dependent on NF-κB [62].

Dendritic cells (DCs), a group of professional antigen-presenting cells, are key members that enable cross talk between the innate and adaptive immune systems. They present an antigen to activate naive lymphocytes and assist in the development of specific adaptive immune responses to pathogens. Hypoxia has been found to play an important role in the maturation and cytokines release of DCs, but the mechanism of the related divergent effects still remains controversial [63]. Studies found that the knockdown of HIF-1α in DCs inhibited their maturation and significantly impaired their capability to stimulate allogeneic T cells, probably because of the reliance on the HIF-controlled glycolysis [64, 65]. In contrast, it is reported that low oxygen tension inhibited the DCs' defense against LPS, but strongly upregulated the production of proinflammatory cytokines in the cells involved [66]. Similar results can be observed in the human antifungal response: hypoxia at the site of *Aspergillus fumigatus* infection inhibited the full activation and function of DCs [67]. These findings suggest that hypoxia may function as a regulator against DCs' mediated immune overreaction.

Lymphocytes are known to be involved in periodontal tissues' health homeostasis, and their functional upset was believed to be associated with periodontal pathogenesis. An HIF-1α deficiency was associated with abnormal B cell development, which led to autoimmunity in a mouse model [68]. A recent study also indicated that T cells' HIF-1α regulation played a critical role in avoiding cardiac damage in diabetic mice [69]. We postulated that a similar protection mechanism may be called to function in diabetic periodontium. Therefore, hypoxia or HIF-1α regulation in DCs and lymphocytes may confer a marked impact on the innate and adaptive cellular immunity in periodontal tissues, with the exact mechanism yet to be elucidated.

5. HIF and epithelial barrier function

The human periodontium is a unique environment for microorganisms. One special characteristic is the nonshedding tooth's hard tissue surface, allowing microorganisms to remain *in situ*. To counter the invasion of possible pathogens, the corresponding epithelial tissues build up an effective barrier against the colonizing microbes [70]. With appropriate daily oral hygiene, the continued host-bacteria interaction maintains the periodontium in health or low grade/subclinical inflammation. Those who have inadequate oral hygiene tip the balance toward a proinflammatory state, resulting in inflammatory responses that present clinically as gingivitis. Due to poor oral hygiene and inherited or acquired risks, approximately 20% of the human population, develop chronic periodontal inflammation with tissue destruction resulting in what is known as periodontitis [71]. Regardless of the host-parasitic interaction outcomes, humans and their complex residential microflora have coevolved over time [72].

TLRs on the periodontal/gingival epithelial cells recognize the conserved molecular patterns on pathogenic bacteria that are also known as PAMP, limiting invasion of the microbes, and help to maintain oral health [73]. Other than providing a physical barrier to the outside world, the skin and mucosal membrane produce a number of antimicrobial peptides (AMPs). The AMPs have a broad activity spectrum against both Gram-negative and Gram-positive bacteria colonization, enveloped viruses, fungi, and even transformed or cancerous cells.

It has become clear that AMPs, such as defensins and the cathelicidins family of peptides—especially LL-37, play important roles independently or together in maintaining oral health, including antimicrobial effects and mediating chemotaxis of the immune cells [74, 75]. Researchers reported that a deficit of cathelicidin allowed infection by *A. actinomycetemcomitans* and the development of severe periodontitis [76].

The epithelial cells in both oral mucosa and the gut are relatively hypoxic [4, 77]. The corresponding oxygen gradient between the epithelium and subepithelial perfusion in turn provides a matching cellular HIF-1α gradient in the tissues involved and perhaps the respective physiological function in cellular homeostasis. In human intestine, when the oxygen supply was impaired due to stasis of the local perfusion, the affected site would be left with increased susceptibility to infection [78]. As such, appropriate adaptive response to hypoxia at the epithelial barriers is vital. HIF-1α functions as an intracellular pO_2 sensor, enabling appropriate adaptive responses for cell survival. Using prolyl hydroxylase inhibitor or AKB-4924, a HIF-1α stabilizing agent, production of cathelicidin and β-defensin in uroepithelial cells was significantly enhanced, and *Escherichia coli* infection was deterred [79]. On the other hand, a deletion of HIF-1α in skin keratinocytes decreased the production of cathelicidin and led to increased susceptibility of infection by a group of *A. Streptococcus* [80]. Naturally occurring low-grade hypoxic reaction and hence HIF-1 accumulation in gut/urogenital/skin epithelia followed by corresponding HIF-1 downstream genes expression were recently postulated to be a key concept that underpin biological barrier function of intestinal epithelium [77, 81]. If in case the same biological process is also in action at the dentogingival junction, HIF-1 would contribute in the periodontal epithelial barrier function that maintains periodontal health and prevents oral pathogenic microorganism invasion.

Besides AMPs, there are also many factors regulated by HIF at the periodontal epithelial barrier. For instance, trefoil factors (TFF), secreted molecules from mucous epithelia, were involved in oral protection against tissue damage and immune response [82, 83]. Their expression was influenced by cellular pO_2 levels. It was reported that HIF-1 mediated the induction of TFF gene expression and provided an adaptive link for the maintenance of the barrier function during hypoxia of gastric/intestinal lining cells [84, 85]. Salivary mucins form a protective layer on the oral surfaces including that of oral sulcular and junctional epithelia, which serve as a physical barrier against bacterial invasion and function as essential antimicrobial macromolecules [86, 87]. Similar to TFF, mucins' production was upregulated in hypoxia [88]. This evidence indicated that the epithelial barrier cells' HIF regulation may constitute an important defense mechanism. Such oral protective machinery could contribute an additional local defense mechanism against periodontal diseases.

6. HIF in the periodontopathogen-host cross talk

Hypoxia is common in the inflammatory microenvironment, and appropriate cellular responses to hypoxia contribute to mucosal defense through the oxygen-sensitive transcription regulator HIF-1α. Hypoxia increases the expression of certain TLRs on human gingival keratinocytes [89], the interaction of low oxygen with appropriate bacteria ligands *in vivo* could potentially enhance the production of cytokines and antimicrobial peptides and thus, in theory, could help to eliminate or reduce the pathogen-related concerns.

The human periodontium is persistently exposed to risks of infection; the source is the commensal and pathogenic oral microorganisms constituting the dental plaque adhering onto teeth. Bacterial components, such as LPS and peptidoglycans, released by bacteria recognized by TLRs on the surface of host cells could instigate the inflammatory reaction cascade [38]. Under steady-state conditions, activation of TLRs by commensal bacteria is critical for the maintenance of oral health [73]. Thus, TLRs provide the first line of defense in periodontal health maintenance. When stimulated, such as via TLRs recognition, PMNs exhibit increased chemotaxis and proinflammatory cytokine production [90].

Our group previously reported that bacterial components may induce HIF-1α accumulation during periodontal disease pathogenesis independent of hypoxia [91]. An immunoprecipitation experiment showed that human gingival fibroblasts' HIF-1α accumulation was induced by LPS in the dose- and time-dependent manner. The accumulation of HIF-1α may be modulated by TLRs and pattern recognition in certain ways, since a TLR4 neutralizing antibody could attenuate such an effect from *E. coli* LPS. Moreover, the expression of TLR4, CD14, and MD-2 in both human gingival keratinocytes and fibroblasts is confirmed, and the TLR4 protein expression in periodontal epithelial compartments appeared different *in vivo*, indicating that LPS sensing in the dentogingival front in health could be heterogeneous in nature [92].

A recent study on oral squamous cell carcinoma provided a novel mechanism of HIF-1 and TLRs' interplay. It was reported that the activation of TLR3 and TLR4 stimulated the expression of HIF-1 through NF-κB, while HIF-1 accumulation increased the expression of TLR3 and TLR4 through direct promoter binding [93]. This observation provided evidence that the TLR3/4-NF-κB pathway may form a positive feedback loop with HIF-1, which theoretically could also happen in the periodontal tissue. Further investigations are needed to confirm such a postulation.

7. HIF and bone homeostasis

HIF appears to play important functional roles in bone homeostasis. The regulatory system seemed complex because HIF is known to stimulate both bone resorption and regeneration, the two essential biological processes in bone homeostasis/repair.

It is reported that a lack of oxygen in periodontal tissues may contribute to alveolar bone resorption and, in theory, accelerated periodontitis [94]. Chromatin immunoprecipitation showed that HIF-1α binds to the receptor activator of the NF-κB ligand (RANKL) promoter region, and mutations of the putative HIF-1α binding site prevented hypoxia-induced RANKL transcriptional promotion, thus suggesting that HIF-1α mediates hypoxia-induced upregulation of RANKL expression and enhanced osteoclastogenesis [95]. Furthermore, it was reported that hypoxia triggered the differentiation of peripheral mononuclear blood cells into functional osteoclasts in a HIF-dependent manner [96].

Conversely, in recent studies, HIF-1α was considered to be a critical mediator of neoangiogenesis required for bone regeneration. Exposure of PDL stem cells to hypoxia improved their osteogenic potential, mineralization and paracrine release, and the mitogen-activated protein kinase kinase/extracellular signal-regulated kinase, and p38 MAPK signaling pathways were involved [97–99]. It was suggested that HIF, HIF mimicking agents, or HIF stabilizing agents were considered triggers for the initiation and promotion of angiogenic-osteogenic coupling [100, 101]. A recent animal study reported new bone and vessels formation induced by the overexpression of HIF-1α via adenovirus, leading to enhanced alveolar bone defect regeneration [102]. A similar result was reported from a study investigating bone loss arrest in ovariectomized C57BL/6 J mice via activated HIF-1α and Wnt/β-catenin signaling pathways [103]. Cementoblastic differentiation of human dental stem cells, a key cellular mechanism concerning periodontal regeneration, was reported to be stimulated by hypoxia in an HIF-1-dependent manner [104].

Taken together, these reports suggested that HIF-1α plays a part in alveolar bone homeostasis, resorption, or periodontal regeneration, while the exact nature of HIF-1α's roles in these processes and the way in which the related pathophysiological processes were regulated warrants further investigations.

8. Conclusions

It seems that tissue/cellular hypoxia, or more specifically, expression of HIF-1α, is involved in periodontal inflammation. HIF-1 not only mediates the host's immune response, providing defense against microbial invaders and maintaining periodontal health, but also could facilitate periodontal-supporting tissue breakdown and, hence, the progression of periodontitis.

Putting all currently available information together, it appears that hypoxia could bring either beneficial or detrimental effects on periodontal health. At the present juncture, we hypothesize that similar to the intestines, a low-grade hypoxia or low level of HIF-1 is expressed in the human periodontium for baseline defense or to act as a surveillance "alarm" against significant invasion or periodontitis. A successful immune response that associates with appropriate HIF-1 mediated biological reactions would result in periodontal health maintenance. Over- or underactivation of the immune system with or without the corresponding dysregulation of HIF-1 biology in tissues as well as alveolar bone, however, could give rise to periodontal tissue damages. We also postulate that other risk indicators related to progression of periodontitis, such as smoking and diabetes mellitus, under the influence of periodontal plaque biofilm, may exert their harmful effects via inappropriate activation of the HIF pathway. Effects of these risks indicators are particular relevant as they often undermine proper periodontal healing/regeneration after therapy [105].

The mechanisms underlying the role of HIF-1 and periodontal defense/pathogenesis, however, remain elusive. Further investigations are, therefore, required in these directions to decipher what leads to the unfavorable immune reactions in periodontal inflammation and the reasons why that came about. Such new knowledge not only fosters the further understanding of human periodontal disease pathogenesis, but may provide novel therapeutic strategies that take advantage of the new understandings of periodontal HIF biology, an important element relevant for periodontal defense and regeneration.

Acknowledgments

The work described in this paper was substantially supported by grants from the Research Grants Council of the Hong Kong Special Administrative Region, China (HKU 17113114), the University of Hong Kong Small Project Funding (201007176307, 201109176129), and Seed Funding (200911159126).

Author details

Xiao Xiao Wang[1], Yu Chen[2,†] and Wai Keung Leung[2,*]

*Address all correspondence to: ewkleung@hku.hk

1 Guanghua School of Stomatology, Provincial Key Laboratory of Stomatology, Sun Yat-sen University, Guangzhou, Guangdong, PR China

2 Faculty of Dentistry, The University of Hong Kong, Hong Kong SAR, PR China

† Current address: Department of Periodontology, Nanjing Stomatology Hospital, Nanjing, Jiangsu Province, PR China

References

[1] Braun RD, Lanzen JL, Snyder SA, Dewhirst MW. Comparison of tumor and normal tissue oxygen tension measurements using OxyLite or microelectrodes in rodents. Am J Physiol Heart Circ Physiol. 2001;280(6):H2533–44.

[2] Yu DY, Cringle SJ. Retinal degeneration and local oxygen metabolism. Exp Eye Res. 2005;80(6):745–51.

[3] Erecinska M, Silver IA. Tissue oxygen tension and brain sensitivity to hypoxia. Respir Physiol. 2001;128(3):263–76.

[4] Mettraux GR, Gusberti FA, Graf H. Oxygen tension (pO_2) in untreated human periodontal pockets. J Periodontol. 1984;55(9):516–21.

[5] Zhu H, Bunn HF. Oxygen sensing and signaling: impact on the regulation of physiologically important genes. Respir Physiol. 1999;115(2):239–47.

[6] Ng KT, Li JP, Ng KM, Tipoe GL, Leung WK, Fung ML. Expression of hypoxia-inducible factor-1alpha in human periodontal tissue. J Periodontol. 2011;82(1):136–41.

[7] Piruat JI, López-Barneo J. Oxygen tension regulates mitochondrial DNA-encoded complex I gene expression. J Biol Chem. 2005;280(52):42676–84.

[8] Semba H, Takeda N, Isagawa T, Sugiura Y, Honda K, Wake M, et al. HIF-1alpha-PDK1 axis-induced active glycolysis plays an essential role in macrophage migratory capacity. Nat Commun. 2016;7:11635.

[9] Wu D, Chen B, Cui F, He X, Wang W, Wang M. Hypoxia-induced microRNA-301b regulates apoptosis by targeting Bim in lung cancer. Cell Prolif. 2016;49(4):476–83.

[10] Li X, Liu Y, Ma H, Guan Y, Cao Y, Tian Y, et al. Enhancement of glucose metabolism via PGC-1alpha participates in the cardioprotection of chronic intermittent hypobaric hypoxia. Front Physiol. 2016;7:219.

[11] Katayama K, Ishida K, Saito M, Koike T, Ogoh S. Hypoxia attenuates cardiopulmonary reflex control of sympathetic nerve activity during mild dynamic leg exercise. Exp Physiol. 2016;101(3):377–86.

[12] Hyun SW, Jung YS. Hypoxia induces FoxO3a-mediated dysfunction of blood-brain barrier. Biochem Biophys Res Commun. 2014;450(4):1638–42.

[13] McDonald PC, Chafe SC, Dedhar S. Overcoming hypoxia-mediated tumor progression: combinatorial approaches targeting pH regulation, angiogenesis and immune dysfunction. Front Cell Dev Biol. 2016;4:27.

[14] Pugh CW. Modulation of the hypoxic response. Adv Exp Med Biol. 2016;903:259–71.

[15] Ward JP. Oxygen sensors in context. Biochim Biophys Acta. 2008;1777(1):1–14.

[16] Yuan C, Wang P, Zhu L, Dissanayaka WL, Green DW, Tong EH, et al. Coculture of stem cells from apical papilla and human umbilical vein endothelial cell under hypoxia

increases the formation of three-dimensional vessel-like structures in vitro. Tissue Eng Part A. 2015;21(5–6):1163–72.

[17] Song ZC, Zhou W, Shu R, Ni J. Hypoxia induces apoptosis and autophagic cell death in human periodontal ligament cells through HIF-1alpha pathway. Cell Prolif. 2012;45(3):239–48.

[18] Teppo S, Sundquist E, Vered M, Holappa H, Parkkisenniemi J, Rinaldi T, et al. The hypoxic tumor microenvironment regulates invasion of aggressive oral carcinoma cells. Exp Cell Res. 2013;319(4):376–89.

[19] Dehne N, Fuhrmann D, Brüne B. Hypoxia-inducible factor (HIF) in hormone signaling during health and disease. Cardiovasc Hematol Agents Med Chem. 2013;11(2):125–35.

[20] Weigent DA. Hypoxia and cytoplasmic alkalinization upregulate growth hormone expression in lymphocytes. Cell Immunol. 2013;282(1):9–16.

[21] Pelosi M, Lazzarano S, Thoms BL, Murphy CL. Parathyroid hormone-related protein is induced by hypoxia and promotes expression of the differentiated phenotype of human articular chondrocytes. Clin Sci (Lond). 2013;125(10):461–70.

[22] Gordon HA, Rovin S, Bruckner G. Blood flow, collagen components of oral tissue and salivary kallikrein in young to senescent, germfree and conventional rats. A study on the etiologic factors of periodontal disease. Gerontology. 1978;24(1):1–11.

[23] Fong GH. Mechanisms of adaptive angiogenesis to tissue hypoxia. Angiogenesis. 2008;11(2):121–40.

[24] Kim JW, Tchernyshyov I, Semenza GL, Dang CV. HIF-1-mediated expression of pyruvate dehydrogenase kinase: a metabolic switch required for cellular adaptation to hypoxia. Cell Metab. 2006;3(3):177–85.

[25] Kojima H, Kobayashi A, Sakurai D, Kanno Y, Hase H, Takahashi R, et al. Differentiation stage-specific requirement in hypoxia-inducible factor-1alpha-regulated glycolytic pathway during murine B cell development in bone marrow. J Immunol. 2010;184(1):154–63.

[26] Phan AT, Goldrath AW. Hypoxia-inducible factors regulate T cell metabolism and function. Mol Immunol. 2015;68(2 Pt C):527–35.

[27] Semenza GL. Oxygen sensing, hypoxia-inducible factors, and disease pathophysiology. Annu Rev Pathol. 2014;9:47–71.

[28] Oliveira RR, Fermiano D, Feres M, Figueiredo LC, Teles FR, Soares GM, et al. Levels of candidate periodontal pathogens in subgingival biofilm. J Dent Res. 2016;95(6):711–8.

[29] Karhausen J, Haase VH, Colgan SP. Inflammatory hypoxia: role of hypoxia-inducible factor. Cell Cycle. 2005;4(2):256–8.

[30] Vasconcelos RC, Costa Ade L, Freitas Rde A, Bezerra BA, Santos BR, Pinto LP, et al. Immunoexpression of HIF-1alpha and VEGF in periodontal disease and healthy gingival tissues. Braz Dent J. 2016;27(2):117–22.

[31] Peyssonnaux C, Datta V, Cramer T, Doedens A, Theodorakis EA, Gallo RL, et al. HIF-1alpha expression regulates the bactericidal capacity of phagocytes. J Clin Invest. Jul 2005;115(7):1806–15.

[32] Dehne N, Brune B. HIF-1 in the inflammatory microenvironment. Exp Cell Res. 2009;315(11):1791–7.

[33] Boronat-Catala M, Catala-Pizarro M, Bagan Sebastian JV. Salivary and crevicular fluid interleukins in gingivitis. J Clin Exp Dent. 2014;6(2):e175–9.

[34] Ozcan E, Saygun NI, Serdar MA, Bengi VU, Kantarci A. Non-surgical periodontal therapy reduces saliva adipokines and matrix metalloproteinases levels in periodontitis. J Periodontol. 2016;87(8):934-43.

[35] Pumklin J, Bhalang K, Pavasant P. Hypoxia enhances the effect of lipopolysaccharide stimulated IL-1beta expression in human periodontal ligament cells. Odontology. 2016;104(3):338-46.

[36] Golz L, Memmert S, Rath-Deschner B, Jager A, Appel T, Baumgarten G, et al. Hypoxia and *P. gingivalis* synergistically induce HIF-1 and NF-kappa B activation in PDL cells and periodontal diseases. Mediators Inflamm. 2015;2015:438085.

[37] Jian C, Li C, Ren Y, He Y, Li Y, Feng X, et al. Hypoxia augments lipopolysaccharide-induced cytokine expression in periodontal ligament cells. Inflammation. 2014;37(5):1413–23.

[38] Mahanonda R, Pichyangkul S. Toll-like receptors and their role in periodontal health and disease. Periodontol 2000. 2007;43:41–55.

[39] Li W, Zhu Y, Singh P, Ajmera DH, Song J, Ji P. Association of common variants in MMPs with periodontitis risk. Dis Markers. 2016;2016:1545974.

[40] Kim YS, Shin SI, Kang KL, Chung JH, Herr Y, Bae WJ, et al. Nicotine and lipopolysaccharide stimulate the production of MMPs and prostaglandin E2 by hypoxia-inducible factor-1alpha up-regulation in human periodontal ligament cells. J Periodontal Res. 2012;47(6):719–28.

[41] Golz L, Memmert S, Rath-Deschner B, Jager A, Appel T, Baumgarten G, et al. LPS from *P. gingivalis* and hypoxia increases oxidative stress in periodontal ligament fibroblasts and contributes to periodontitis. Mediators Inflamm. 2014;2014:986264.

[42] Duscher D, Maan ZN, Whittam AJ, Sorkin M, Hu MS, Walmsley GG, et al. Fibroblast-specific deletion of hypoxia inducible factor-1 critically impairs murine cutaneous neovascularization and wound healing. Plast Reconstr Surg. 2015;136(5):1004–13.

[43] Tong C, Hao H, Xia L, Liu J, Ti D, Dong L, et al. Hypoxia pretreatment of bone marrow-derived mesenchymal stem cells seeded in a collagen-chitosan sponge scaffold promotes skin wound healing in diabetic rats with hindlimb ischemia. Wound Repair Regen. 2016;24(1):45–56.

[44] Zhu T, Park HC, Son KM, Yang HC. Effects of dimethyloxalylglycine on wound healing of palatal mucosa in a rat model. BMC Oral Health. 2015;15:60.

[45] Huang J, Liu L, Feng M, An S, Zhou M, Li Z, et al. Effect of $CoCl_2$ on fracture repair in a rat model of bone fracture. Mol Med Rep. 2015;12(4):5951–6.

[46] Fujio M, Xing Z, Sharabi N, Xue Y, Yamamoto A, Hibi H, et al. Conditioned media from hypoxic-cultured human dental pulp cells promotes bone healing during distraction osteogenesis. J Tissue Eng Regen Med. 2015; DOI: 10.1002/term.2109

[47] Nizet V, Johnson RS. Interdependence of hypoxic and innate immune responses. Nat Rev Immunol. 2009;9(9):609–17.

[48] Sitkovsky M, Lukashev D. Regulation of immune cells by local-tissue oxygen tension: HIF1 alpha and adenosine receptors. Nat Rev Immunol. 2005;5(9):712–21.

[49] Huang X, Yu T, Ma C, Wang Y, Xie B, Xuan D, et al. Macrophages play a key role in the obesity induced periodontal innate immune dysfunction via NLRP3 pathway. J Periodontol. 2016;23:1–18; DOI: 10.1902/jop.2016.160102

[50] Hajishengallis G, Chavakis T, Hajishengallis E, Lambris JD. Neutrophil homeostasis and inflammation: novel paradigms from studying periodontitis. J Leukoc Biol. 2015;98(4):539–48.

[51] Walmsley SR, Cadwallader KA, Chilvers ER. The role of HIF-1alpha in myeloid cell inflammation. Trends Immunol. 2005;26(8):434–9.

[52] Gale DP, Maxwell PH. The role of HIF in immunity. Int J Biochem Cell Biol. 2010;42(4):486–94.

[53] Lall H, Coughlan K, Sumbayev VV. HIF-1alpha protein is an essential factor for protection of myeloid cells against LPS-induced depletion of ATP and apoptosis that supports toll-like receptor 4-mediated production of IL-6. Mol Immunol. 2008;45(11):3045–9.

[54] Frede S, Stockmann C, Winning S, Freitag P, Fandrey J. Hypoxia-inducible factor (HIF) 1alpha accumulation and HIF target gene expression are impaired after induction of endotoxin tolerance. J Immunol. 2009;182(10):6470–6.

[55] Frede S, Stockmann C, Freitag P, Fandrey J. Bacterial lipopolysaccharide induces HIF-1 activation in human monocytes via p44/42 MAPK and NF-kappa B. Biochem J. 2006;396(3):517–27.

[56] Kong T, Eltzschig HK, Karhausen J, Colgan SP, Shelley CS. Leukocyte adhesion during hypoxia is mediated by HIF-1-dependent induction of beta 2 integrin gene expression. Proc Natl Acad Sci U S A. 2004;101(28):10440–5.

[57] Massena S, Christoffersson G, Vagesjo E, Seignez C, Gustafsson K, Binet F, et al. Identification and characterization of VEGF-A-responsive neutrophils expressing CD49d, VEGFR1, and CXCR4 in mice and humans. Blood. 2015;126(17):2016–26.

[58] Walmsley SR, Print C, Farahi N, Peyssonnaux C, Johnson RS, Cramer T, et al. Hypoxia-induced neutrophil survival is mediated by HIF-1alpha-dependent NF-kappa B activity. J Exp Med. 2005;201(1):105–15.

[59] Rius J, Guma M, Schachtrup C, Akassoglou K, Zinkernagel AS, Nizet V, et al. NF-kappa B links innate immunity to the hypoxic response through transcriptional regulation of HIF-1alpha. Nature. 2008;453(7196):807–11.

[60] Belaiba RS, Bonello S, Zahringer C, Schmidt S, Hess J, Kietzmann T, et al. Hypoxia up-regulates hypoxia-inducible factor-1alpha transcription by involving phosphatidylinositol 3-kinase and nuclear factor kappa B in pulmonary artery smooth muscle cells. Mol Biol Cell. 2007;18(12):4691–7.

[61] Yeramian A, Santacana M, Sorolla A, Llobet D, Encinas M, Velasco A, et al. Nuclear factor-kappa B2/p100 promotes endometrial carcinoma cell survival under hypoxia in a HIF-1alpha independent manner. Lab Invest. 2011;91(6):859–71.

[62] Bonello S, Zahringer C, BelAiba RS, Djordjevic T, Hess J, Michiels C, et al. Reactive oxygen species activate the HIF-1alpha promoter via a functional NFkappa B site. Arterioscler Thromb Vasc Biol. 2007;27(4):755–61.

[63] O'Neill LA, Pearce EJ. Immunometabolism governs dendritic cell and macrophage function. J Exp Med. 2016;213(1):15–23.

[64] Fluck K, Breves G, Fandrey J, Winning S. Hypoxia-inducible factor 1 in dendritic cells is crucial for the activation of protective regulatory T cells in murine colitis. Mucosal Immunol. 2016;9(2):379–90.

[65] Jantsch J, Chakravortty D, Turza N, Prechtel AT, Buchholz B, Gerlach RG, et al. Hypoxia and hypoxia-inducible factor-1 alpha modulate lipopolysaccharide-induced dendritic cell activation and function. J Immunol. 2008;180(7):4697–705.

[66] Mancino A, Schioppa T, Larghi P, Pasqualini F, Nebuloni M, Chen IH, et al. Divergent effects of hypoxia on dendritic cell functions. Blood. 2008;112(9):3723–34.

[67] Fliesser M, Wallstein M, Kurzai O, Einsele H, Loffler J. Hypoxia attenuates anti-*Aspergillus fumigatus* immune responses initiated by human dendritic cells. Mycoses. 2016;59(8):503–8.

[68] Kojima H, Gu H, Nomura S, Caldwell CC, Kobata T, Carmeliet P, et al. Abnormal B lymphocyte development and autoimmunity in hypoxia-inducible factor 1 alpha-deficient chimeric mice. Proc Natl Acad Sci U S A. 2002;99(4):2170–4.

[69] Lin Y, Tang Y, Wang F. The protective effect of HIF-1alpha in T lymphocytes on cardiac damage in diabetic mice. Ann Clin Lab Sci. 2016;46(1):32–43.

[70] Groeger SE, Meyle J. Epithelial barrier and oral bacterial infection. Periodontol 2000. 2015;69(1):46–67.

[71] Ng SKS, Leung WK. A community study on the relationship between stress, coping, affective dispositions and periodontal attachment loss. Community Dent Oral Epidemiol. 2006;34(4):252–66.

[72] Ostaff MJ, Stange EF, Wehkamp J. Antimicrobial peptides and gut microbiota in homeostasis and pathology. EMBO Mol Med. 2013;5(10):1465–83.

[73] Hans M, Hans VM. Toll-like receptors and their dual role in periodontitis: a review. J Oral Sci. 2011;53(3):263–71.

[74] Greer A, Zenobia C, Darveau RP. Defensins and LL-37: a review of function in the gingival epithelium. Periodontol 2000. 2013;63(1):67–79.

[75] Turkoglu O, Emingil G, Kutukculer N, Atilla G. Gingival crevicular fluid levels of cathelicidin LL-37 and interleukin-18 in patients with chronic periodontitis. J Periodontol. 2009;80(6):969–76.

[76] Eick S, Puklo M, Adamowicz K, Kantyka T, Hiemstra P, Stennicke H, et al. Lack of cathelicidin processing in Papillon-Lefevre syndrome patients reveals essential role of LL-37 in periodontal homeostasis. Orphanet J Rare Dis. 2014;9:148.

[77] Colgan SP, Taylor CT. Hypoxia: an alarm signal during intestinal inflammation. Nat Rev Gastroenterol Hepatol. 2010;7(5):281–287.

[78] Szabo S. "Gastric cytoprotection" is still relevant. J Gastroenterol Hepatol. 2014;29(Suppl 4):124–32.

[79] Lin AE, Beasley FC, Olson J, Keller N, Shalwitz RA, Hannan TJ, et al. Role of hypoxia inducible factor-1 alpha (HIF-1α) in innate defense against uropathogenic *Escherichia coli* infection. PLoS Pathog. 2015;11(4):e1004818.

[80] Peyssonnaux C, Boutin AT, Zinkernagel AS, Datta V, Nizet V, Johnson RS. Critical role of HIF-1alpha in keratinocyte defense against bacterial infection. J Invest Dermatol. 2008;128(8):1964–8.

[81] Shehade H, Oldenhove G, Moser M. Hypoxia in the intestine or solid tumors: a beneficial or deleterious alarm signal? Eur J Immunol. 2014;44(9):2550–7.

[82] Choudhary A, Smitha CN, Suresh DK. Trefoils: an unexplored natural protective shield of oral cavity. J Oral Biol Craniofac Res. 2015;5(3):226–31.

[83] Chaiyarit P, Chayasadom A, Wara-Aswapati N, Hormdee D, Sittisomwong S, Nakaresisoon S, et al. Trefoil factors in saliva and gingival tissues of patients with chronic periodontitis. J Periodontol. 2012;83(9):1129–38.

[84] Hernandez C, Santamatilde E, McCreath KJ, Cervera AM, Diez I, Ortiz-Masia D, et al. Induction of trefoil factor (TFF)1, TFF2 and TFF3 by hypoxia is mediated by hypoxia inducible factor-1: implications for gastric mucosal healing. Br J Pharmacol. 2009;156(2):262–72.

[85] Furuta GT, Turner JR, Taylor CT, Hershberg RM, Comerford K, Narravula S, et al. Hypoxia-inducible factor 1-dependent induction of intestinal trefoil factor protects barrier function during hypoxia. J Exp Med. 2001;193(9):1027–34.

[86] Kejriwal S, Bhandary R, Thomas B, Kumari S. Estimation of levels of salivary mucin, amylase and total protein in gingivitis and chronic periodontitis patients. J Clin Diagn Res. 2014;8(10):ZC56–60.

[87] Sanchez GA, Miozza VA, Delgado A, Busch L. Relationship between salivary mucin or amylase and the periodontal status. Oral Dis. 2013;19(6):585–91.

[88] Zhou X, Tu J, Li Q, Kolosov VP, Perelman JM. Hypoxia induces mucin expression and secretion in human bronchial epithelial cells. Transl Res. 2012;160(6):419–27.

[89] Chen Y. Hypoxia and *E. coli* LPS-induced periodontal resident cells PAMP expressions: implication for periodontitis pathogenesis. Ph. D. Dissertation, The University of Hong Kong, 2015.

[90] Alvarez ME, Fuxman Bass JI, Geffner JR, Fernandez Calotti PX, Costas M, Coso OA, et al. Neutrophil signaling pathways activated by bacterial DNA stimulation. J Immunol. 2006;177(6):4037–46.

[91] Li JP, Li FY, Xu A, Cheng B, Tsao SW, Fung ML, et al. Lipopolysaccharide and hypoxia-induced HIF-1 activation in human gingival fibroblasts. J Periodontol. 2012;83(6):816–24.

[92] Li JP, Chen Y, Ng CH, Fung ML, Xu A, Cheng B, et al. Differential expression of toll-like receptor 4 in healthy and diseased human gingiva. J Periodontal Res. 2014;49(6):845–54.

[93] Shengwei H, Wenguang X, Zhiyong W, Xiaofeng Q, Yufeng W, Yanhong N, et al. Crosstalk between the HIF-1 and toll-like receptor/nuclear factor-κB pathways in the oral squamous cell carcinoma microenvironment. Oncotarget. 2016; DOI: 10.18632/oncotarget.9329

[94] Yu XJ, Xiao CJ, Du YM, Liu S, Du Y, Li S. Effect of hypoxia on the expression of RANKL/OPG in human periodontal ligament cells in vitro. Int J Clin Exp Pathol. 2015;8(10):12929–35.

[95] Park HJ, Baek KH, Lee HL, Kwon A, Hwang HR, Qadir AS, et al. Hypoxia inducible factor-1α directly induces the expression of receptor activator of nuclear factor-κB ligand in periodontal ligament fibroblasts. Mol Cells. 2011;31(6):573–8.

[96] Dandajena TC, Ihnat MA, Disch B, Thorpe J, Currier GF. Hypoxia triggers a HIF-mediated differentiation of peripheral blood mononuclear cells into osteoclasts. Orthod Craniofac Res. 2012;15(1):1–9.

[97] Wu Y, Yang Y, Yang P, Gu Y, Zhao Z, Tan L, et al. The osteogenic differentiation of PDLSCs is mediated through MEK/ERK and p38 MAPK signalling under hypoxia. Arch Oral Biol. 2013;58(10):1357–68.

[98] Wu Y, Cao H, Yang Y, Zhou Y, Gu Y, Zhao X, et al. Effects of vascular endothelial cells on osteogenic differentiation of noncontact co-cultured periodontal ligament stem cells under hypoxia. J Periodontal Res. 2013;48(1):52–65.

[99] Zhao L, Wu Y, Tan L, Xu Z, Wang J, Zhao Z, et al. Coculture with endothelial cells enhances osteogenic differentiation of periodontal ligament stem cells via cyclooxygenase-2/prostaglandin E2/vascular endothelial growth factor signaling under hypoxia. J Periodontol. 2013;84(12):1847–57.

[100] Mamalis AA, Cochran DL. The therapeutic potential of oxygen tension manipulation via hypoxia inducible factors and mimicking agents in guided bone regeneration. A review.. Arch Oral Biol. 2011;56(12):1466–75.

[101] Ding H, Gao YS, Wang Y, Hu C, Sun Y, Zhang C. Dimethyloxaloylglycine increases the bone healing capacity of adipose-derived stem cells by promoting osteogenic differentiation and angiogenic potential. Stem Cells Dev. 2014;23(9):990–1000.

[102] Zhang Y, Huang J, Wang C, Hu C, Li G, Xu L. Application of HIF-1alpha by gene therapy enhances angiogenesis and osteogenesis in alveolar bone defect regeneration. J Gene Med. 2016;18(4–6):57–64.

[103] Peng J, Lai ZG, Fang ZL, Xing S, Hui K, Hao C, et al. Dimethyloxalylglycine prevents bone loss in ovariectomized C57BL/6 J mice through enhanced angiogenesis and osteogenesis. PLoS One. 2014;9(11):e112744.

[104] Choi H, Jin H, Kim JY, Lim KT, Choung HW, Park JY, et al. Hypoxia promotes CEMP1 expression and induces cementoblastic differentiation of human dental stem cells in an HIF-1-dependent manner. Tissue Eng Part A. 2014;20(1–2):410–23.

[105] Grossi SG, Skrepcinski FB, DeCaro T, Zambon JJ, Cummins D, Genco RJ. Response to periodontal therapy in diabetics and smokers. J Periodontol. 1996;67(10 Suppl):1094–102.

Permissions

List of Contributors

Ana Marina Andrei, Anca Berbecaru-Iovan, Felix Rareş Ioan Din-Anghel, Camelia Elena Stănciulescu, Sorin Berbecaru-Iovan, Ileana Monica Baniţă and Cătălina Gabriela Pisoschi
University of Medicine and Pharmacy of Craiova, Craiova, Dolj County, Romania

Dominga Iacobazzi, Massimo Caputo and Mohamed T Ghorbel
University of Bristol, School of Clinical Sciences, Bristol Heart Institute, Bristol, UK

Deepak Bhatia and Shahrzad Movafagh
Bernard J Dunn School of Pharmacy, Shenandoah University, VA, USA

Mohammad Sanaei Ardekani
Kidney and Hypertension Specialists, VA, USA

Qiwen Shi
Collaborative Innovation Center of Yangtza River Delta Region Green Pharmaceuticals, Zhejiang University of Technology, Hangzhou, Zhejiang

Sandeep Artham
Program in Clinical and Experimental Therapeutics, College of Pharmacy, University of Georgia and the Charlie Norwood VA Medical Center, Augusta, GA, USA

Payaningal R. Somanath
Program in Clinical and Experimental Therapeutics, College of Pharmacy, University of Georgia and the Charlie Norwood VA Medical Center, Augusta, GA, USA
Department of Medicine, Vascular Biology Center and Cancer Center, Augusta University, Augusta, GA, USA

Raja El Hasnaoui-Saadani
Research center-College of Medicine- Princess Nourah bint Abdulrahmane University, Riyadh, Saudi Arabia

Bernardo J. Krause
Division of Pediatrics, Department of Neonatology, The Pontifical Catholic University of Chile, Santiago, Chile

Paola Casanello
Division of Pediatrics, Department of Neonatology, The Pontifical Catholic University of Chile, Santiago, Chile
Division of Obstetrics & Gynecology, School of Medicine, The Pontifical Catholic University of Chile, Santiago, Chile

Emilio A. Herrera
Pathophysiology Program, Biomedical Sciences Institute (ICBM), Faculty of Medicine, University of Chile, Santiago, Chile

Markus Mandl and Reinhard Depping
Institute of Physiology, Center for Structural and Cell Biology in Medicine, University of Luebeck, Luebeck, Germany

Xiao Xiao Wang
Guanghua School of Stomatology, Provincial Key Laboratory of Stomatology, Sun Yat-sen University, Guangzhou, Guangdong, PR China

Yu Chen and Wai Keung Leung
Faculty of Dentistry, The University of Hong Kong, Hong Kong SAR, PR China

Index

A

Acute Kidney Injury, 43, 61-62, 64, 80-81

Acute Lung Injury, 43, 84-86, 99, 101-102

Acute Respiratory Distress Syndrome, 84, 98

Adipocyte Hypertrophy, 4, 7-8

Adiponectin, 5-8, 11, 15, 18, 21, 25

Adipose Tissue Hypoxia, 1-3, 7-9, 11, 17, 20, 23

Allograft Rejection, 43, 67

Alzheimer's Disease, 43-44, 67, 70-71, 73-75

Amyotrophic Lateral Sclerosis, 46, 68-69, 72-74

Angiogenesis, 1, 3, 8-9, 13-16, 18-22, 24-25, 36, 38, 43, 50-51, 56, 60, 79, 88, 97-98, 104-111, 113-118, 135-136, 156, 158, 165-166, 172

Angiogenin, 49, 69-70

Anti-inflammatory Adipocytokines, 1-2

Arnt, 140-154

Atherosclerosis, 9, 131, 136

B

Body Mass Index, 2, 17

Brown Adipose Tissue, 1-4, 25

C

Cardiac Function, 104, 107, 109, 118

Cardiac Surgery, 29, 34-35, 41-42

Cardiopulmonary Bypass, 27, 32-34, 37, 40-42

Cardiovascular Diseases, 5, 28, 39, 43-44, 116, 121

Cerebral Blood Flow, 44, 104-105, 111, 114-116, 118

Cerebral Stroke, 1-2

Cerebrovascular Diseases, 43

Chronic Anemia, 104-106, 108-112, 114

Chronic Hypoxia, 7, 24, 28-33, 35-36, 38, 40, 42, 47, 54, 62, 69, 75, 80, 85, 87-88, 98-100, 104-111, 114-116, 119, 121-122, 124, 133

Chronic Inflammation, 1, 3, 11, 18, 157

Chronic Obstructive Pulmonary Disease, 43, 95

Chronic Periodontitis, 155, 170

Congenital Heart Disease, 27, 29-30, 36-40, 42

Connective Tissue Growth Factor, 12, 90

Cyanosis, 27, 30-31, 33, 40-42

E

Erythropoiesis, 43, 50, 82

Erythropoietin, 30, 51, 64-65, 72-74, 82, 105, 108, 110, 113-114, 116-120

Extracellular Matrix, 5, 23, 27, 30, 94, 158

F

Fetal Growth Restriction, 121-124, 132-134

G

Glutathione Peroxidase, 29, 124

H

Heart Failure, 28, 30, 38, 43, 117

Hepatocellular Carcinoma, 148-150, 154

Hypercaloric Diet, 8, 12, 14

Hyperoxia, 7, 9, 11, 115

Hyperplasia, 8, 14

Hypoxia, 1-4, 7-9, 11-18, 20-21, 23-25, 27-33, 35-40, 42-82, 84-124, 127-130, 133-134, 136-148, 151-172

Hypoxia-inducible Factor, 8, 25, 36, 38, 42, 50, 99-102, 104, 113-114, 117, 119, 155-156, 165-170

Hypoxic Signaling, 43, 55-56, 58, 61

I

Inflammatory Bowel Disease, 43, 55-56, 58, 78-79, 93, 97

Insulin Resistance, 6, 8-9, 11-13, 17-20, 22

Interstitial Lung Disease, 84

Ischemic Heart Disease, 1-2, 30

L

Leptin, 4-9, 11, 15, 20-22, 88, 99

Lipolysis, 5, 8-9, 11, 21

M

Macrophage Infiltration, 3-4

Macrophage Migration Inhibitory Factor, 4, 7

Matrix Metalloproteinases, 4, 6, 8, 12, 30, 60, 158, 167

Metabolic Syndrome, 1-2, 5, 7, 9-10, 15-16, 121, 128, 131

Migration Inhibitory Factor, 4, 7

Myocardial Infarction, 28, 39

Myocardial Protection, 27, 35, 37, 41-42

N

Neprilysin, 45, 68, 75

Neurodegenerative Disease, 43

Neuropathy, 47-48

Normoxia, 7-9, 11, 14, 31, 55, 111, 119-120, 143

O

Obstructive Sleep Apnea, 14, 43

Omentin, 5-6, 20

Oxygen Homeostasis, 104-105, 153

P

Parkinson's Disease, 43-45, 68-70, 72, 74-75

Periodontal Ligament, 157, 166-167, 171

Periodontal Pocket, 155-156

Prostaglandins, 5, 64, 81, 95

Pulmonary Arterial Hypertension, 31, 38-39, 84, 87, 98-100

Pulmonary Disease, 28, 43, 95

Pulmonary Hypertension, 28, 30, 38-39, 43, 85, 88, 99-100, 107, 111, 137, 139

R

Reactive Oxygen Species, 3, 21-22, 27, 29, 69, 75, 82, 86, 100, 124, 148, 158, 169

Reoxygenation Injury, 27, 32-34, 36, 40-42

Rheumatoid Arthritis, 43, 55, 60, 79-80

Right Ventricular Hypertrophy, 30, 88, 117

S

Stromo-vascular Fraction, 1-2, 4-5, 7

T

Tetralogy of Fallot, 28-29, 37-40, 42

Toll-like Receptor, 9, 158, 168, 171

Transforming Growth Factor, 4, 6, 57, 90, 100-101, 160

Traumatic Brain Injury, 44, 48, 70, 74, 114, 139

V

Vascular Endothelial Growth Factor, 4, 6-7, 30, 39, 72-73, 78-80, 85, 98-99, 104-105, 113, 152, 171

Vascular Permeability, 6, 15, 20, 85-86, 92, 98, 106

W

White Adipose Tissue, 1-2, 4, 13, 16, 18

Wound Resolution, 84

X

Xenograft Model, 149, 150

www.ingramcontent.com/pod-product-compliance
Lightning Source LLC
Chambersburg PA
CBHW050500200326
41458CB00014B/5244